Paleo Autoimmune Protocol

Paleo Autoimmune Protocol

Paleo Recipes and Meal Plan to Heal Your Body

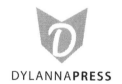

DYLANNA**PRESS**

First edition: 2014

Disclaimer/Limit of Liability

This book is for informational purposes only. The views expressed are those of the author alone, and should not be taken as expert, legal, or medical advice. The reader is responsible for his or her own actions.

Every attempt has been made to verify the accuracy of the information in this publication. However, neither the author nor the publisher assumes any responsibility for errors, omissions, or contrary interpretation of the material contained herein.

This book is not intended to provide medical advice. Please see your health care professional before embarking on any new diet or exercise program. The reader should regularly consult a physician in matters relating to his/her health and particularly with respect to any symptoms that may require diagnosis or medical attention.

CONTENTS

Introduction 3

Autoimmune Disease and Diet 4

What Is a Leaky Gut? (And how to tell if you have one)...... 6

What Is the Paleo Autoimmune Protocol? 9

Getting Started 10

Phase 1, Elimination 10

Phase 2, Reintroduction 20

FAQs 25

Factors Other than Diet to Consider 29

Meal Plan 31

Part II - Recipes

Breakfast 39

Appetizers, Salads, and Snacks 53

Soups and Stews 71

Meat and Poultry 83

Seafood 107

Side Dishes 119

Sweets and Treats 137

Resources 141

Index 143

INTRODUCTION

IF YOU ARE reading this book, then you are probably suffering from one of the many types of autoimmune disease. First, be assured that you are not alone. Autoimmune diseases have increased to epidemic proportions and there are currently an estimated 50 million Americans with an autoimmune issue. Why has autoimmunity become such a huge problem for so many people? Scientific research on the subject all seems to lead back to the same source—today's modern diet and stress-filled lifestyle has wreaked havoc on our digestive systems, leading to systemic inflammation, pain, and in many people, chronic autoimmune diseases such as celiac disease, multiple sclerosis, rheumatoid arthritis, psoriasis, and numerous other conditions.

The good news is that there are ways that you can address the symptoms and root causes of autoimmune disease naturally, through diet, without having to rely on medications or an array of supplements. By making dietary changes and eliminating the foods that cause digestive problems and a leaky gut, you can heal your immune system and rebuild your health.

This book is intended to provide an overview of the Paleo Autoimmune Protocol (AIP) and help guide you through the process of transforming your diet and regaining control over your health. The book contains details about the AIP, its guidelines, and its many benefits. Also included is a meal plan to make it easier to stick to the Autoimmune Protocol, as well as detailed shopping lists, and many delicious, easy-to-prepare, AIP-compliant recipes. Following the Paleo Autoimmune Protocol isn't easy, it requires willpower and 100 percent commitment for a minimum of 30 days, but the benefits are enormous and potentially life changing. This book attempts to make it as easy as possible for you to learn about and implement the AIP.

AUTOIMMUNE DISEASE AND DIET

There are many different types of autoimmune disease and they are becoming more and more common. The exact reasons for the increase are not entirely clear but research has shown a strong connection between the food we put into our bodies and the symptoms of autoimmunity.

Most, if not all, autoimmune diseases have a common factor and that is chronic inflammation. These diseases occur when the immune system begins to attack the body's own proteins, mistaking them for foreign invaders. Instead of releasing chemicals in response to toxins and trauma, the body will start releasing chemicals against its own cells. Because of markers known as antibodies, the immune response attacks the body's own cells, starting inflammation.

People with an autoimmune disease may experience chronic symptoms or they may have flares. During flares, the immune response is strong enough to damage the mistaken enemy. As a result, the system that is under attack (the joints in rheumatoid arthritis, or organs in lupus, for example) start to show signs of serious damage. Even during less active days, someone with an autoimmune disease may experience constant inflammation, as the mistaken irritant is always present.

Common Autoimmune Disorders and the Cells They Attack:

- *Multiple Sclerosis:* Brain and spinal cord cells are mistaken as enemies.

- *Crohn's Disease*: Inflammation causes damage to the lining of the intestines.

- *Lupus:* Cells from multiple areas such as the skin, heart, vascular system, kidneys, nervous system, muscles, and connective tissues are mistaken and trigger an autoimmune attack.

- *Hashimoto's Thyroiditis:* The cells of the thyroid are attacked, resulting in thyroid failure.

- *Rheumatoid Arthritis:* Connective tissues within the joints are the target in this inflammatory condition.

- *Type 1 Diabetes:* Insulin-producing pancreas cells are destroyed, resulting in the inability to correctly regulate blood sugar.

- *Celiac Disease:* Gluten triggers an autoimmune attack against villi cells, an important part of the intestines.

There are many more autoimmune diseases—such as psoriasis, Grave's disease, and ulcerative colitis—all affecting different parts of the body. While the severity and specifics of the diseases may vary, they often overlap. It is even common for people with autoimmune diseases to be diagnosed with more than one. Because of this phenomenon, inflammation for these groups of people can easily be widespread throughout the body.

There are many factors that can cause autoimmune disorders, genetic susceptibility being an important one, but diet certainly has a prominent role. One leading theory on the link between diet and autoimmunity has to do with what is called a *leaky gut*.

WHAT IS A LEAKY GUT? (AND HOW TO TELL IF YOU HAVE ONE)

The science behind the autoimmune protocol is based on the theory that autoimmune diseases result from a problem with intestinal permeability, otherwise known as leaky gut. In a healthy gut, the permeability of the intestinal wall is well-regulated and allows only very small molecules, such as nutrients, to pass through. In sensitive individuals, irritants in the diet, such as gluten, can cause the tight junctions in the intestinal lining to loosen and let larger molecules—such as toxins, undigested food, and bacteria—escape from the gut and travel to other parts of the body through the bloodstream. Once these particles are recognized by the body's immune system they are identified as "invaders" and the immune response kicks in, releasing antibodies and causing systemic inflammation.

Gluten, while a common culprit, is not the only cause of a leaky gut. Depending on the individual, there are many other potential causes including dairy, sugar, alcohol, environmental toxins, antibiotics, stress, and aging. The Autoimmune Paleo Protocol is designed to remove as many of these potential irritants as possible from your diet and therefore give your body and gut a chance to heal. Depending on the extent of the current damage to your intestines, this could be as little as 30 days to perhaps several months or longer.

SIGNS OF A LEAKY GUT

Any of the following are indications that you may be suffering from a leaky gut:

- Digestive problems, including gas, bloating, cramps, diarrhea, IBS

- Allergies, both seasonal and food

- Asthma

- Skin problems, including acne, eczema, rosacea

- Mood disorders, including anxiety, depression, and ADD

- Fibromyalgia

- Candida overgrowth

- Autoimmune diseases, including celiac disease, rheumatoid arthritis, lupus, psoriasis, multiple sclerosis

- Hormonal imbalances

- Joint pain

WHAT IS THE PALEO AUTOIMMUNE PROTOCOL?

THE AUTOIMMUNE Paleo Protocol, or AIP, was originally created by Robb Wolf and Dr. Loren Cordain and further researched and developed by Sarah Ballantyne. It is an elimination diet designed to reduce inflammation in your body, improve digestive health, and heal a leaky gut. When following the AIP you remove the foods that cause irritation and trigger autoimmune antibodies. Removing these irritants allows your gut, and therefore your body, to heal. Once your gut has healed and autoimmune antibodies are no longer being released there should be a dramatic reduction in symptoms.

This is a restrictive, intensive protocol that is meant to be followed for a *temporary* period—anywhere from a minimum of 30 days to perhaps several months, depending on your specific issues and response to the protocol. Once your gut has healed, then you will be able to slowly reintroduce foods back into your diet, and gauge your body's reaction to them. Any foods that trigger an autoimmune response will need to be permanently removed from your diet.

This section has provided just a brief overview of the science behind the protocol, for a more in-depth look we recommend consulting some of the books provided in the references section, such as *The Paleo Approach* by Sarah Ballantyne.

GETTING STARTED

The Autoimmune Paleo Protocol is basically an elimination diet and as such it requires 100 percent commitment in order to be effective. This means there are no "cheat" days and even minor slip-ups can send you back to square one. This is not written to be discouraging, but instead to make you aware that committing to this is going to require, well, commitment. Psyching yourself up mentally and being prepared are very important to the success of this protocol. Just remember that the results, in terms of the incredible benefits to your health, can be truly life-changing and well worth the effort needed to succeed. Also keep in mind that you are not meant to stay on the Autoimmune Protocol forever. The majority of foods on the "Foods to Avoid" list can be reintroduced into your diet. See the section on Phase 2, Reintroduction for more about the best way to add foods back into your diet.

One of the ways to help ensure your success in following the protocol is to plan ahead. Set a date for yourself and then stick to it. Enlist support for family and friends. Plan out your meals and stock your kitchen. In order to help you get organized and plan ahead we've included a detailed grocery list as well as a 14-day meal plan to help you get prepared.

PHASE 1, ELIMINATION

The first part of the protocol involves eliminating any potentially irritating foods from your diet and allowing your body and gut time to heal. This can take anywhere from a minimum of 30 days to several months or perhaps more. It is recommended that you stay on the restricted protocol until your symptoms subside and you feel significantly better.

Below is a list of foods that need to be avoided on the Autoimmune Paleo Protocol. This is followed by a list of foods that can be eaten while on the protocol.

FOODS TO AVOID ON THE PALEO AUTOIMMUNE PROTOCOL

GRAINS (ALL TYPES)
- barley
- buckwheat
- bulgur
- corn
- farro
- millet
- oats
- quinoa
- rice
- rye
- sorghum
- spelt
- wheat

DAIRY AND EGGS
- butter
- cheese
- cream
- eggs

- ghee
- milk
- yogurt

LEGUMES AND BEANS

- beans of all types
- peas
- chickpeas
- lentils
- peanuts
- soybeans

NIGHTSHADE VEGETABLES

- cayenne
- eggplant
- goji berry
- paprika
- peppers (all types)
- potatoes
- pepper-based spices
- tomatoes
- tomatillo

NUTS AND SEEDS (ALL TYPES)

OILS

- corn
- cottonseed
- canola
- grapeseed
- margarine
- palm kernel
- peanut

- safflower
- shortening
- soybean
- sunflower
- vegetable

CHOCOLATE

COFFEE

ALCOHOL

PROCESSED FOODS

SWEETENERS
- agave
- sugar
- stevia

NON-STEROIDAL ANTI-INFLAMMATORY DRUGS (NSAIDS)
- aspirin
- ibuprofen
- naproxen

Okay, after reading that list it may seem like there's nothing left to eat on the Paleo Autoimmune Protocol! But don't worry, there is plenty of delicious food that is still allowed.

FOODS TO ENJOY ON THE PALEO AUTOIMMUNE PROTOCOL

VEGETABLES (ALL TYPES EXCEPT FOR NIGHTSHADES)

- artichokes
- arugula
- asparagus
- avocado
- beets
- bok choy
- broccoli
- Brussels sprouts
- cabbage
- carrots
- cauliflower
- celery
- collard greens
- cucumber
- endive
- fennel
- kale
- kudzu
- leeks
- lettuce
- maca
- mushrooms (all types)
- okra
- onions
- parsley
- parsnips
- pumpkin

- radicchio
- radish
- rutabaga
- seaweed/sea vegetables
- shallots
- spinach
- squash (all types)
- sweet potato
- Swiss chard
- turnips
- wasabi
- water chestnuts
- watercress
- yams
- zucchini

FRUITS

- apples
- apricot
- avocado
- banana
- berries
- blackberries
- blueberries
- cantaloupe
- cherries
- citrus fruits
- coconut
- cranberries
- dates
- figs
- grapefruit

- grapes
- guava
- kiwis
- lemon
- lime
- mango
- olives
- oranges
- papaya
- peaches
- pears
- pineapple
- plums
- pomegranates
- raspberries
- rhubarb
- strawberries
- watermelon

MEATS

It is important to buy good-quality meats. Opt for grass-fed and/or wild whenever possible. Avoid processed and cured meats such as hot dogs.

- beef
- bison
- chicken
- deer
- duck
- goat
- lamb
- organ meats/offal – heart, liver, kidney, etc.

- pheasant
- pork
- quail
- rabbit
- turkey
- veal
- wild game

SEAFOOD AND FISH

- anchovies
- bass
- clams
- cod
- crab
- fish – all types
- grouper
- haddock
- halibut
- lobster
- mackerel
- mahi mahi
- mussels
- octopus
- oysters
- red snapper
- salmon
- sardines
- scallops
- shrimp
- sole
- squid
- tilapia

- trout
- tuna

FATS AND OILS
- avocado oil
- bacon fat
- coconut oil
- lard
- olive oil
- palm oil

FERMENTED FOODS
- kefir – water, coconut
- kimchi
- kombucha
- sauerkraut

HERBS, SEASONINGS, AND MISCELLANEOUS ITEMS
- agar agar
- arrowroot powder
- baking soda
- basil
- bay
- capers
- carob powder
- chamomile
- chervil
- chives
- cilantro
- cinnamon
- cloves
- coconut aminos
- coconut flour

- dill
- fennel
- fish sauce
- garlic
- gelatin
- ginger
- honey (limited)
- lavender
- lemon balm
- lemongrass
- marjoram
- mint
- oregano
- rosemary
- saffron
- sage
- salt (Himalyan or sea salt)
- tapioca powder
- tarragon
- thyme
- turmeric

BEVERAGES

- coconut milk
- coconut water
- herbal tea – chamomile, dandelion root, ginger, hibiscus, lavender, mint, rose hip, etc.
- kefir – water, coconut
- kombucha
- vegetable juice
- water – carbonated, mineral, soda, sparkling

As you can see there are still a lot of things you can eat while following this plan!

PHASE 2, REINTRODUCTION

As stated earlier, the AIP is not meant to last forever. After a certain period of time, be it 30 days, 60 days, or perhaps longer, it will be time to start reintroducing foods back into your diet. This is important for a couple of reasons. One being that the Autoimmune Protocol is a very restrictive diet and most people will not be able to keep to such restrictions forever. In addition, variety is an important part of a well-balanced, nutritious diet and so it is a good idea to have as many nutritious food options as possible available to choose from.

So where do you start? Do you just go back to eating your normal diet as soon as the 30 days are over? Absolutely not. The key is to reintroduce foods slowly, testing your body's reaction to them individually, and then deciding whether your body tolerates them well and if they can be included in your personal, individualized diet. In addition, there are certain foods that should be eliminated permanently (see table below).

Many people, after following the AIP for a while and seeing a big improvement in their health, are hesitant to start reintroducing foods back into their diets, afraid it will cause them to relapse back to where they were before. However, it's a mistake to try and stay on the strict Autoimmune Paleo Protocol forever. It is too restrictive nutritionally, as well as psychologically, to stay on indefinitely.

The timing of reintroduction is a personal decision. It is suggested to wait until you start to see improvement in your symptoms. For some this may be as soon as 30 days, for others it could be several months or longer.

Once you have made the decision to start reintroducing foods back into your diet it is very important not to rush the reintroduction process. Allow a minimum of two to three months to complete it. The reintroduction phase is a process of trial and error where you will discover if any of the foods that are added back in are causing your symptoms to flair.

Start with one food at a time, choosing those that are least likely to be causing any issues. In the beginning, start with just a small portion of the food. Eat that food at least twice on two consecutive days. Watch yourself closely for any negative reactions. It may take up to 72 hours for any reactions to occur. Types of negative reactions may include an increase in your autoimmune disease symptoms, aches and pains, fatigue, headache, rash, digestive problems, moodiness, or sleep difficulties. If any of these symptoms occur, then eliminate the offending food from your diet permanently. If you do not experience any negative symptoms after a week of eating that food then that food is safe to add back into your diet. One thing to keep in mind during this process, however, is that not all foods will elicit an immediate strong negative reaction. Some responses may start off very small and not be noticeable right away but may build up over the course of several days. This is why it is extremely important not to rush when reintroducing foods. Take your time and be sure there is no reaction before adding another food.

Allow a couple of days to pass before attempting to reintroduce another food. Keep repeating this process until you have successfully either permanently eliminated or reintroduced all of the desired foods back into your diet. At the end of the process you should have a personalized diet tailor made to keep you in the best state of health.

It is a good idea to keep a record, such as journal, during this period, making note of how you feel after each successive food is reintroduced.

ORDER OF REINTRODUCTION

The following lists the recommended order of reintroducing foods back into your diet. It is best to start with those foods least likely to cause problems and work your way up to those more prone to causing issues.

FIRST FOODS TO REINTRODUCE
- Egg yolks
- Ghee
- Seeds, seed-based spices, seed oils
- Nuts

NEXT FOODS TO TRY
- Butter
- Goat dairy products – yogurt, cheese, milk
- Cow dairy products – yogurt, cheese, milk
- Coffee
- Cocoa/chocolate
- Alcohol – small quantities

FOODS TO REINTRODUCE LAST
- Egg whites
- Nightshades – potatoes, peppers and pepper-based spices, eggplant, tomatoes, goji berries, etc.

FOODS TO ELIMINATE PERMANENTLY FROM YOUR DIET
- Processed foods
- Sugar and non-nutritive sweeteners
- Grains

- Refined oils
- Legumes (including soy and peanuts)

SUMMARY OF THE AIP

- Eliminate all of the foods from the not allowed list from your diet for 30-60 days (perhaps more depending on your body's response).

- Eat high-quality, nutrient dense foods from the allowed list of foods.

- Reintroduce foods slowly, one a time, gauging your body's reaction to them. If you experience an increase in your symptoms or other negative side effects, then remove that food from your diet permanently.

- Look at other areas in your life, outside of diet, that may be affecting your health status such as inadequate sleep and/or stress overload. Take steps to correct these areas such as making sure you are getting a minimum of 7-8 hours' sleep per night and making time for exercise and other stress-relieving activities such as yoga and meditation.

The ultimate goal here is to create a personalized diet for your unique body and sensitivities that will be sustainable and provide long-term health benefits.

FAQs

Do I have to start all over again if I slip up and eat something from the not allowed list?

In a word, yes. Unfortunately, that is the nature of an elimination diet. That being said, there are many people who favor a more gradual approach to the Autoimmune Paleo Protocol and easing into it (for example, by cutting out only gluten to begin with or transitioning to a Paleo diet for a few months) may be the best way for many. In fact, for some, just modifying their diet enough to be Paleo may be enough to send their symptoms into remission. But for many others this won't be enough and following the strict AIP will be necessary, with no cheating, in order to see results.

While this may seem tough, and it is, try and remember that it is not forever and focus your mind on the incredible benefits you will receive if you stick with it.

Who should consider trying the Paleo Autoimmune Protocol?

Anyone who is currently dealing with autoimmunity issues should consider going on the AIP. Specifically, it has been shown to be beneficial for the following conditions:

- celiac disease

- Crohn's disease

- eczema

- Grave's disease

- Hashimoto's disease

- lupus

- multiple sclerosis

- psoriasis

- rheumatoid arthritis

- ulcerative colitis

How much fruit is allowed on the Autoimmune Protocol?

Since fruit contains a significant amount of natural sugar many people wonder about eating too much fruit while on the AIP. Fruit is not generally restricted while on the protocol and since it is full of fiber, vitamins, and other nutrients, it is not something that should be avoided.

However, if blood glucose regulation is a concern, then you may want to limit yourself to 2-3 servings of fruit per day.

I am concerned about losing too much weight while on the Autoimmune Protocol, any suggestions?

The best way to avoid losing too much weight is to make sure you are eating plenty of healthy fats, starchy vegetables, and other calorie-dense foods. Eating plenty of avocados, sweet potatoes, beets, coconut oil/milk, and fruit and vegetable juices daily is an excellent way of making sure you do not lose too much weight.

What can I eat for breakfast if eggs and dairy aren't allowed?

For many people breakfast is the most challenging meal of the day when following the Autoimmune Protocol. If you are used to eating eggs or yogurt for breakfast, then it may be hard to figure out how to substitute for these foods. One thing that may help is to stop thinking of only traditional breakfast foods as being appropriate to eat in the morning. There's no hard and fast rule that says you can't enjoy lunch or dinner foods at breakfast. A nice warm bowl of chicken soup may be just the thing to start your day.

Check out the meal plans and recipes for ideas on what you can have for breakfast.

What about medications, should they be discontinued while on the protocol?

No, it is not advised that any medications be stopped while on the Autoimmune Protocol. It is recommended that you consult with your health care professional before starting the AIP and as your symptoms improve it is best to consult with your doctor about how and when to reduce or eliminate medications.

How do I handle going out to eat while on the protocol?

This is a tough one. The easiest answer is to say don't go out while on the AIP. However, this is not realistic and there are times when you'll want or need to have a meal out of the house. Here are some general tips for ordering in restaurants:

- Order a salad (no tomatoes) and ask for olive oil and vinegar on the side as dressing.

- Order plain grilled meat, chicken, or fish with veggies on the side.

- Read all menu items carefully and ask your server how the food is prepared.

FACTORS OTHER THAN DIET TO CONSIDER

While diet is probably the most important factor in your health there are several other components that can be equally influential.

Sleep. Getting adequate sleep is one of the best things you can do for your body. Most people require a minimum of 7-8 hours of sleep per night. You may need more than this if you are battling autoimmune disease. Without enough sleep it will be very hard for your body to heal itself. Make sleep a priority.

Stress. Too much or chronic stress can wreak havoc on your digestive system, gut health, and hormone levels. It is important not to take on more than you can handle. Find ways to reduce the stress in your life and incorporate stress-relieving activities such as yoga, tai chi, meditation, and deep breathing exercises.

Exercise. Staying fit and getting regular exercise are a big part of staying healthy. However, if you are suffering from fatigue, joint pain, or other symptoms that can interfere with getting regular exercise this may be a challenge. Try doing gentle stretching exercises, yoga, or taking walks.

Supplements. Some people find that changing their diet alone isn't enough. In this case, there are some supplements that may help boost your body's healing process. It is recommended that you consult with a functional medicine doctor or holistic practitioner to determine which supplements would be best for your particular situation. Some to consider are digestive enzymes, probiotics, omega-3s, L-glutamine, magnesium, vitamin C, and collagen.

Support. Trying to go on the Autoimmune Protocol without support from your loved ones is going to be difficult. Sit down and talk to them about the protocol and ways they can help and support you. Finding support from others who are also in the same situation as you can also be an enormous help. The Internet is a great place to find others who are on the same journey.

MEAL PLAN

WEEK ONE

Day One

- Breakfast: *Banana-Apple Smoothie with Greens*
- Lunch: *Greens Chicken Salad with Root Vegetable Dressing*
- Dinner: *Pan-Seared Salmon on Baby Arugula*
- Snack: *Guacamole with raw vegetables*

Day Two

- Breakfast: *Spinach and Sausage Breakfast Stir-Fry*
- Lunch: *Easy Chicken, Kale, and Carrot Soup*
- Dinner: *Glazed Pork Roast with Carrots, Parsnips, and Pears*
- Snack: *Apple or Pear*

Day Three

- Breakfast: *Cinnamon-Squash Breakfast Bowl*
- Lunch: *Leftover Pork with Mixed Vegetable and Fruit Salad*
- Dinner: *Beef and Veggie Stir-Fry with Ginger-Orange Sauce*
- Snack: *Hot Baked Cinnamon Apples*

Day Four

- Breakfast: *Kale and Mango Smoothie*
- Lunch: *Cream of Chicken Soup*
- Dinner: *Grilled Whitefish with Oregano; Roasted Balsamic Vegetables*
- Snacks: *Coconut Milk Yogurt topped with berries*

Day Five

- Breakfast: *Broiled Grapefruit*
- Lunch: *Portobello Burger*
- Dinner: *Turkey and Orange Stir-Fry*
- Snacks: *Piece of fruit*

Day Six

- Breakfast: *Easy Bacon, Mushroom, and Kale Skillet*

Breakfast

- Lunch: *Salmon Salad with Fresh Dill and Veggies*

- Dinner: *Fried Chicken with Avocado and Red Onion Salsa*

- Snacks: *Chopped Turnip Appetizer*

Day Seven

- Breakfast: *Banana-Pear Breakfast Medley*

- Lunch: *Asian Shrimp and Coconut Soup*

- Dinner: *Grilled Balsamic Lamb Chops*

- Snacks: *Black Olive Tapenade with Tuna*

WEEK TWO

Day One

- Breakfast: *Avocado-Berry Smoothie*

- Lunch: *Cream of Broccoli Soup*

- Dinner: *Asian Chicken Lettuce Wraps*

- Snacks: *Kale Chips*

Day Two

- Breakfast: *Coconut Milk Yogurt topped with berries*

- Lunch: *Mixed green salad topped with avocado and tuna*

- Dinner: *Paleo Chicken in a Pot*
- Snacks: *Vegetable chips*

Day Three

- Breakfast: *Paleo Breakfast Sausage, fresh fruit*
- Lunch: *Spinach Salad with Apple*
- Dinner: *Grilled Marinated Tuna in Foil with Onions*
- Snacks: *Guacamole and veggies*

Day Four

- Breakfast: *Coconut-Banana "Oatmeal"*
- Lunch: *Fruit Carrot Soup, green salad*
- Dinner: *Grilled grass-fed beef; Broccoli with Ginger*
- Snacks: *Kale and Mango Smoothie*

Day Five

- Breakfast: *Easy Bacon, Mushroom and Kale Skillet*
- Lunch: *Lemony Garlic Shrimp over Zoodles*
- Dinner: *Chicken, Bacon, and Mushroom Skewers, Cauli-Rice*
- Snacks: *Piece of fruit*

Day Six

- Breakfast: *Broiled Grapefruit, Bacon*

- Lunch: *Grilled Chicken Salad with Mango and Avocado*

- Dinner: *Tender Grilled Pork Tenderloin, Roasted Sweet Potato with Rosemary*

- Snacks: *Kale Chips*

Day Seven

- Breakfast: *Banana-Apple Smoothie with Greens*

- Lunch: *Smoked Salmon and Sweet-Potato Hash*

- Dinner: *Chicken Piccata*

- Snacks: *Coconut Date Bites*

Part II
Recipes

Breakfast

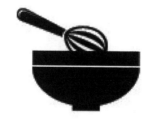

CARROT, CABBAGE, AND PEACH SMOOTHIE

Servings: 4

Ingredients:

- 1 cup grapes
- 1 cup frozen peaches, sliced
- 3/4 cup cabbage, chopped
- 1 large carrot
- 1/4 cup ice cubes, or as desired
- 1/4 cup water, or as desired

Directions:

1. In a blender, combine all ingredients. Blend until smooth.

2. Serve in 4 tall glasses.

BANANA-APPLE SMOOTHIE WITH GREENS

Servings: 4

Ingredients:

- **1 ripe banana**
- **1 apple, cored and peeled**
- **1 carrot, chopped**
- **2 cups filtered water**
- **1 tablespoon raw honey**
- **1 cup whole coconut milk**
- **4 cups greens—romaine, spinach, chard, kale, collards, parsley etc.**

Directions:

1. In a food processor, combine all ingredients except the greens. Process until smooth.
2. Mix in four cups of mixed greens and blend until smooth.

COCONUT-BANANA "OATMEAL"

*Servings:*1

Ingredients:

- **1 banana**
- **2 tablespoons coconut butter**
- **½ teaspoon cinnamon**
- **Sea salt**
- **Blueberries for topping**
-

Directions:

1. In a small bowl, mash banana. Add salt and cinnamon.

2. In a saucepan, warm coconut butter over low heat. (Alternative-ly, place in microwave-safe bowl and heat for about 30 seconds.)

3. Add coconut butter to banana mixture and stir.

4. Top with blueberries or other favorite fruit.

KALE AND MANGO SMOOTHIE

Servings: 2

Ingredients:

- **2 cups kale**
- **1 mango, peeled and diced**
- **1 kiwi, peeled and diced**
- **1 cup coconut milk**
- **Juice of ½ lime**

Directions:

Add all ingredients to blender. Process until smooth.

Serve in tall glasses.

SPINACH AND SAUSAGE BREAKFAST STIR-FRY

Servings: 2

Ingredients:

- **1 tablespoon coconut oil**
- **½ yellow onion, diced**
- **½ pound sausage**
- **4 cups spinach**

Directions:

1. In a skillet, heat coconut oil over medium heat.

2. Add onions and sauté for 2-3 minutes until translucent.

3. Add sausage and cook until browned, stirring frequently.

4. Add spinach, reduce heat to low, and continue to cook, stirring occasionally, until spinach is wilted, about 4-5 minutes.

5. Serve hot.

EASY BACON, MUSHROOM, AND KALE SKILLET BREAKFAST

Servings: 2

Ingredients:

- **4-6 strips bacon**
- **½ onion, chopped**
- **1 cup mushrooms, stems removed, sliced in half**
- **2 cups kale, washed and trimmed**
- **½ teaspoon thyme**
- **Pinch of Himalayan salt**

Directions:

1. Place bacon strips in large skillet. Cook over medium heat until desired crispiness (about 10-12 minutes). Remove bacon strips from pan and set aside. Leave 2 tablespoons bacon grease in pan, drain off any extra.

2. Add onion to skillet and cooking over medium heat, stirring, for 2-3 minutes. Add mushrooms and continue to cook, stirring occasionally, until mushrooms are soft, about 3-4 minutes.

3. Add kale to skillet, and continue to sauté, stirring occasionally, until kale has wilted, about 3-4 minutes.

4. Season with thyme and salt. Serve vegetable mixture hot with bacon strips on the side.

AVOCADO-BERRY SMOOTHIE

Servings: 2

Ingredients:

- **1 avocado, peeled, pitted, cubed**
- **½ cup coconut milk**
- **1 cup fresh strawberries (could also use fro zen)**
- **1 cup frozen raspberries**
- **Juice of ½ lime**

Directions:

1. Place all ingredients into a blender. Process until smooth.
2. Serve in tall glasses.

CINNAMON-SQUASH BREAKFAST BOWL

Serves: 2

Ingredients:

- **1 acorn squash, cut in half, seeds removed**
- **¼ cup coconut milk**
- **1 tablespoon cinnamon**
- **1 apple, peeled and chopped**

Directions:

1. Place acorn squash cut side down in shallow baking pan filled with ½-inch water. Bake in 350 degree oven for 30 minutes or until squash is tender. (Alternatively, wrap each half of squash in microwave-safe plastic wrap and place on plate. Cook in microwave for about 5 minutes or until cooked through.)

2. Let squash cool slightly and then scoop out squash. Puree in food processor or mash by hand with potato masher.

3. Place squash in bowl and add coconut milk and cinnamon. Stir to mix.

4. Top with chopped apples and serve.

PALEO BREAKFAST SAUSAGE

Servings: Makes 8 patties

Ingredients:

- **1 pound ground lean pork**
- **2 teaspoons fresh sage leaves, finely chopped**
- **1 teaspoon fresh thyme, finely chopped**
- **1/4 teaspoon fresh rosemary, chopped**
- **1 tablespoon olive oil**

Directions:

1. In a large bowl, combine all ingredients. Manually mix until well blended. Form 8 patties.

2. In a medium non-stick pan heat oil over medium heat. Cook patties in batches for about 9 minutes on one side then another 6 minutes on the other side or until well browned.

COCONUT MILK YOGURT

Servings: 8

Ingredients:

- **2 13.5 ounce cans coconut milk, full-fat**
- **1 teaspoon gelatin**
- **2 probiotic capsules or one packet yogurt starter**
- **1 large mason jar**

Directions:

1. Pour coconut milk into saucepan and heat gently until it reaches 115 degrees. You will need a candy thermometer to test temperature.

2. Remove from heat and add gelatin. Stir to mix.

3. Open probiotic capsules and sprinkle into milk, or add yogurt starter. Mix well.

4. Pour into sterile glass jar with lid (such as mason jar).

5. Place jar in unheated oven with the oven light on. Close oven door and let the jar sit in the unheated oven for 24 hours. (Alternatively, place the jar in an insulated cooler filled with hot water or wrap the jar in heating pad.) The key is to keep the temperature between 108 and 112 degrees during the incubation process.

6. After 24 hours, mix the yogurt with a spoon and then place in refrigerator for 6-8 hours.

BROILED GRAPEFRUIT

Servings: 1

Ingredients:

- **1 grapefruit, cut in half**
- **½ teaspoon cinnamon**
- **1 teaspoon honey or maple syrup (optional)**

Directions:

1. Using a sharp knife, cut around the edges of the grapefruit and then inside the grapefruit sections, separating the fruit from the rind.

2. Line a broiling pan with parchment paper or foil. Place grapefruit on pan, cut side up. Sprinkle with cinnamon and drizzle with honey or maple syrup.

3. Put under broiler for 3-5 minutes. Serve warm.

BANANA-PEAR BREAKFAST MEDLEY

Servings: 2

Ingredients:

- **1 ripe banana**
- **1 large ripe pear**
- **½ teaspoon cinnamon**
- **Juice from ½ lime**

Directions:

1. Peel banana and slice into round pieces, place in bowl. Peel pear and cut into small chunks, place in bowl with banana. Sprinkle with cinnamon and mix to coat. Add lime juice and mix again. Let marinate for 10 minutes before serving.

Appetizers, Salads, and Snacks

BLACK OLIVE TAPENADE WITH TUNA

Servings: 4-6

Ingredients:

- **3 garlic cloves**
- **1 cup small black olives, drained**
- **1/4 cup capers, rinsed, drained**
- **6 ounces tuna**
- **4 ounces anchovies, drained**
- **1/4 cup plus 2 teaspoons olive oil (divided)**

Directions:

1. In a food processor, combine olives and garlic, pulse to chop. Add in tuna, capers, anchovies, and 1/4 cup olive oil; process until pureed.

2. Scrape and transfer into a bowl. Pour in remaining olive oil without stirring.

3. Cover with plastic wrap and chill for about 6 hours to overnight. It can last for two weeks chilled in an airtight container.

4. Mix well before serving. Serve with crudités.

CHOPPED TURNIP APPETIZER

Servings: 10

Ingredients:

- **1 rutabaga, peeled and chopped**
- **1 turnip, peeled and chopped**
- **1/4 cup olive oil, more as needed**
- **1 small onion, chopped**
- **1 clove garlic, minced**
- **Black pepper, to taste**

Directions:

1. In a food processor set at high, process rutabaga and turnip, adding olive oil while mixing, until smooth.

2. Combine in garlic and onions, process for about 4 minutes until very smooth. Add more oil to desired consistency. Season with pepper.

KALE AND ORANGE SALAD WITH CRAN-BERRY VINAIGRETTE

Servings: 4 to 6

Ingredients:

- **5 ounces mature curly kale leaves, trimmed, coarsely chopped**
- **1 medium navel orange, peeled, sliced coarsely**
- **1/2 cup fresh cranberries, rinsed, picked over, finely chopped**
- **2 tablespoons red wine vinegar**
- **1 tablespoons cranberry juice**
- **4 tablespoons extra-virgin olive oil**
- **2 teaspoons fresh ginger, peeled, finely grated**
- **Sea salt and black pepper, to taste**

Directions:

1. In a salad bowl, mix honey, vinegar, and cranberry juice until well blended. Stir in cranberries and ginger. Add a little salt and pepper.

2. Add in kale and orange slices, toss well to coat. Cover and chill for at least 15 minutes to an hour before serving.

GREENS CHICKEN SALAD WITH ROOT VEGETABLE DRESSING

Servings: 4

Ingredients:

For the Salad

- 2 cups (1/2-inch) skinless chicken breast, cooked, diced
- 1 head romaine lettuce, chopped
- 1 head radicchio, chopped
- 1 Belgian endive, chopped
- 1/2 cup Roasted Root Vegetable Dressing

For Roasted Root Vegetable Dressing (Makes about 2 1/2 cups)

- 2 medium parsnips, peeled and cubed
- 2 medium carrots, peeled and cubed
- 1 large shallot, quartered
- 1 1/3 cups low-sodium chicken broth
- 1/3 cup plus 2 tablespoon extra-virgin olive oil
- 1/4 cup unsweetened apple juice concentrate
- 1 teaspoon pure maple syrup
- 3 tablespoon apple cider vinegar
- 3/4 teaspoon sea salt
- 1/4 teaspoon freshly ground black pepper

Directions:

1. Preheat oven to 425°F.

2. On a rimmed baking sheet, combine root vegetables and drizzle 2 tablespoons of oil. Toss to coat. Evenly spread and roast for about 30 minutes or until tender. Cool.

3. In a food processor, combine cooled roasted vegetables with the rest of the ingredients. Process until smooth.

4. In a large bowl, combine all ingredients for the salad. Add the dressing and toss to coat.

COCONUT LIME FRUIT SALAD

Servings: 4

Ingredients:

- **2 cups strawberries, halved**
- **2 cups honeydew melon, chopped into cubes**
- **1 mango, chopped**
- **1⁄4 cup coconut milk**
- **4 teaspoon fresh lime juice**
- **2 teaspoon fresh basil, chopped**
- **1⁄2 teaspoon raw honey**
- **Dash of sea salt**

Directions:

1. In a salad bowl, combine the fruits. In another bowl, whisk coconut milk with lime juice, honey and basil. Season with some salt. Pour dressing onto the fruits. Toss to blend.

SPINACH SALAD WITH APPLE

Servings: 4

Ingredients:

- **3 tablespoon extra-virgin olive oil**
- **1 1/2 tablespoons cider vinegar**
- **1 tablespoon horseradish, prepared**
- **1/2 teaspoon sea salt**
- **1 red apple, halved, cored, sliced**
- **1/2 cup pomegranate seeds**
- **1/4 cup red onion, thinly sliced**
- **3/4 pound fresh baby spinach, rinsed, stems cut, leaves torn**

Directions:

1. In a salad bowl, combine oil, vinegar, and horseradish, whisk to blend. Season with salt. Mix in apple and onions, toss to combine. Put inside the fridge for 30 minutes.

2. Add spinach, mix, and serve.

MIXED VEGETABLE AND FRUIT SALAD

Servings: 4

Ingredients:

- 1 apple, skin on, diced
- 1 cup cantaloupe, diced
- 1/2 English cucumber, skin on
- 1 orange, zested and flesh cut up, diced
- 1 lime, zested and juiced
- Cinnamon
- Sea salt and black pepper, to taste
- Fresh basil leaves, as garnish

Directions:

1. Into a bowl, combine all ingredients. Mix to incorporate. Season with salt and pepper to taste.

2. Scoop into serving bowls, garnish with additional cinnamon and basil leaves.

CRAB STUFFED MUSHROOMS

Servings: 4

Ingredients:

- 2 cups crab meat
- 10 ounces package frozen spinach, chopped, drained
- 1 1/2 pound Portobello mushrooms, stems chopped, tops reserved
- 1/4 cup onions, chopped
- 2 cloves garlic, minced
- 1/2 teaspoon dried basil, crushed
- 1/2 dried oregano, crushed
- 1/4 teaspoon ground ginger
- 1/4 cup white wine
- 1 tablespoon fresh squeezed lemon juice

Directions:

1. Preheat oven to 425 °F.
2. In a non-stick pan, cook mushroom stems, onions, garlic, lemon juice, and white wine for about 5 minutes over medium flame until tender. Add spinach, cook over low heat until most of the liquid is gone. Mix in oregano, basil, and ginger into spinach mixture; continue cooking for several seconds. Add crab meat, slowly mix until cooked through.
3. Scoop crab meat mixture into mushroom tops. Place on lightly greased baking pan and bake for about 15 minutes or until tender.

SALMON SALAD WITH FRESH DILL AND VEGGIES

Servings: 4

Ingredients:

- **2 cans wild salmon**
- **2 cucumbers, diced**
- **1 onion, chopped**
- **1 avocado, diced**
- **6 tablespoon extra-virgin olive oil**
- **2 lemons, juiced**
- **2 tablespoon fresh dill, chopped**
- **Salt and pepper, to taste**
- **Lettuce leaves, for serving**

Directions:

1. Drain the extra liquid from canned wild salmon and transfer to a bowl. Add in cucumbers, onions, avocado, extra-virgin olive oil, lemon juice, fresh dill, salt, and pepper.

2. Mix them well. Cover the salad and refrigerate for at least 2-3 hours. Place the chilled salmon salad on lettuce leaves and serve.

GRILLED CHICKEN SALAD WITH MANGO AND AVOCADO

Servings: 4

Ingredients:

- **2 tablespoons olive oil, divided**
- **Juice of 1 lime**
- **1 tablespoon honey**
- **1 teaspoon fresh ginger, grated**
- **4 skinless, boneless chicken breasts**
- **2 mangoes, peeled and diced**
- **2 avocados, peeled and diced**
- **8 cups mixed salad greens**
- **1 tablespoon balsamic vinegar**

Directions:

1. In a small bowl, combine 1 tablespoon olive oil, lime, honey, and ginger.

2. Place chicken on plate and brush each side with oil mixture. Grill chicken until cooked through, flipping once and brushing with oil mixture. Slice cooked chicken into strips.

3. Add salad greens to large salad bowl. Add sliced chicken, mango, and avocado. Drizzle with remaining olive oil and balsamic vinegar.

GUACAMOLE

Servings: 4

Ingredients:

- **2 avocados, mashed**
- **¼ white onion, minced**
- **2 garlic cloves, minced**
- **¼ teaspoon garlic powder**
- **Juice of ½ a lime**
- **Salt and pepper, to taste**

Directions:

1. Mix all ingredients in a small bowl. Whisk until well blended.

KALE CHIPS

Servings: 6

Ingredients:

- **1 large bunch kale**
- **2 tablespoons olive oil**
- **1 ½ teaspoons sea salt**

Directions:

1. Preheat oven to 350 degrees Fahrenheit. Line cookie sheet with parchment paper.

2. Cut stems from kale. Wash and thoroughly dry kale leaves.

3. Spread kale out on baking sheet in single layer. Drizzle with olive oil and season with salt.

4. Bake until edges are browned, about 10-12 minutes.

STRAWBERRY SALAD

Servings: 2

Ingredients:

- **1 pint strawberries, washed and cut in thirds**
- **3 cups mesclun greens**
- **1 celery stalk, chopped**
- **1 fennel bulb, chopped**
- **¼ balsamic vinegar**
- **3 tablespoons extra-virgin olive oil**
- **Freshly ground black pepper, to taste**

Directions:

1. Add strawberries, mesclun greens, celery, and fennel to salad bowl.
2. In a small bowl, whisk together vinegar, oil, and pepper. Pour dressing over salad. Toss to coat.

RAW BROCCOLI SALAD

Servings: 2

Ingredients:

- **3 cups broccoli, washed and chopped into small florets (1/2-inch pieces)**
- **3 cloves garlic, minced**
- **3 tablespoons fresh cilantro, chopped fine**
- **¼ cup extra-virgin olive oil**
- **Juice from 1 lemon**
- **½ teaspoon sea salt**

Directions:

1. Place broccoli in large bowl. Add the remaining ingredients and mix well. Cover and refrigerate for at least one hour to allow broccoli to marinate.

BLUEBERRY-MANGO-PINEAPPLE SALAD

Servings: 4

Ingredients:

- **1 ½ cups fresh pineapple chunks**
- **1 mango, peeled and cut into cubes**
- **1 cup fresh blueberries**
- **¼ large red onion, finely chopped**
- **Juice of 1 lime**

Directions:

1. Combine pineapple, mango, blueberries, and onion in bowl. Pour lime juice over fruit and mix well. Allow to marinate in refrigerator for an hour before serving.

ZUCCHINI PESTO

Servings: 4 cups

Ingredients:

- **2 pounds zucchini**
- **¼ cup olive oil**
- **3 garlic cloves, minced**
- **1 shallot, minced**
- **Sea salt and freshly ground black pepper**

Directions:

1. Coarsely grate zucchini. Place in colander and allow to drain for several minutes.

2. Heat olive oil in a large pot over medium heat. Add garlic and shallot and sauté for 2-3 minutes. Add zucchini and cook for 5-6 minutes or until zucchini is very soft and tender. Remove pan from heat.

3. Using an immersion blender or food processor, process mixture until it reaches a spreadable consistency. Add a little more olive oil if needed. Season with salt and pepper.

4. Can be stored in refrigerator for 2-3 weeks.

Soups and Stews

BONE BROTH

Servings: 6-8

Ingredients:

- **2 ½ - 3 pounds of bones**
- **1 onion, peeled and chopped**
- **1 large carrot, peeled and chopped**
- **3 stalks celery, diced**
- **2 cloves garlic, peeled and chopped**
- **3 tablespoons apple cider vinegar**

Directions:

1. Add all ingredients to large pot. Cover with water and bring to boil. Reduce heat and simmer, covered for at least 6-8 hours.

2. Using a slotted spoon, remove bones and vegetable pieces from broth. Pour broth through mesh strainer to remove any remaining pieces.

3. Broth can be eaten at once or stored in the refrigerator for up to a week.

SHITAKE SOUP WITH SQUASH AND MUSTARD GREENS

Servings: 6-8

Ingredients:

- **15 dried shiitake mushrooms, soaked in boil ing water**
- **12 cups vegetable stock**
- **1/2 small butternut squash, peeled, seeded, cubed**
- **3 tablespoons coconut aminos**
- **1 red onion, quartered and sliced in thin rings**
- **2 large garlic cloves, finely chopped**
- **1 large rosemary sprig**
- **4 large mustard greens, stems removed and coarsely chopped**

Directions:

1. In a large pot, bring broth to boil over high heat. Add in squash, lower heat, cover and simmer.
2. Meanwhile, soak mushrooms in water for 15 minutes, press out absorbed liquid, and pour together with soak water in the pot. Trim soft mushrooms and cut in strips. Mix in the pot.
3. Mix in the remaining ingredients, except for the greens. Continue simmering until squash is tender.
4. Stir in chopped greens and allow several seconds to wilt and turn bright green. Pull pan off heat and serve in bowls at once.

PUMPKIN AND BACON SOUP

Servings: 2

Ingredients:

- **4 slices streaky bacon**
- **1/2 large pumpkin, peeled, seeded, cubed**
- **1 large white onion, finely chopped**
- **2 cloves garlic, minced**
- **1 tablespoon fresh thyme**
- **2 cups chicken broth**

Directions:

1. In a pan, brown bacon over medium high flame. Transfer onto a chopping board, reserving the generated grease. Chop bacon into 1-inch pieces.

2. In the same pan with bacon grease, add the onion and garlic; fry for about 5 minutes over low heat.

3. Add the pumpkin cubes along with the stock. Bring to a boil and let simmer for about 25 minutes.

4. Transfer mixture into a blender and puree until smooth. Pour back into the pot, mix in thyme and bacon. Serve immediately.

CREAM OF CHICKEN SOUP

Servings: 6

Ingredients:

- 1/2 cup coconut oil
- 2 stalks celery, finely diced
- 2 medium carrots, finely diced
- 6 cups chicken broth
- 1/2 cup arrowroot dissolved in 1/2 cup cold water
- 1 teaspoon dried parsley
- 1/2 teaspoon dried thyme
- 1 bay leaf
- 1 teaspoon salt
- 3 cups cooked chicken, cubed
- 1 1/2 cups coconut milk

Directions:

1. In a large pot, heat oil over medium heat; cook carrots and celery for about 10 minutes, stirring occasionally, until tender. Add broth and arrowroot along with bay leaf, parsley, thyme, and salt. Cook while stirring until thickened.

2. Lower the heat and bring to a slow boil; cook for about 15 minutes. Mix in coconut milk and chicken and cook for several minutes until heated through. Adjust desired consistency by adding more broth or water.

FRUITY CARROT SOUP

Servings: 4

Ingredients:

- **2 tablespoon coconut oil**
- **1 small onion, peeled and chopped**
- **5 large carrots, chopped**
- **1 green apple, chopped**
- **½ ounces fresh ginger, chopped**
- **⅓ cup orange juice**
- **1 cup coconut milk**
- **2 cups chicken stock**
- **fresh lime, as garnish**

Directions:

1. In a large pan, heat oil over medium high heat. Cook onion, apples, and carrots for about 5 minutes or until tender. Add ginger, orange juice, coconut milk and chicken stock. Transfer mixture into a food processor, process until pureed. Work in batches if needed.

2. Transfer back into the pan and. Serve garnished with fresh lime.

PURPLE SWEET POTATO SOUP

Servings: 4

Ingredients:

- **1/2 tablespoon olive oil**
- **1/2 of an onion, chopped**
- **1 1/2 pounds purple sweet potato, peeled, chopped**
- **4 cups vegetable broth**
- **1/2 teaspoon sea salt or to taste**
- **1/4 cup coconut milk**

Directions:

1. In a saucepan, heat oil over medium high flame. Add onions and cook for about 5 minutes or until just softened. Add sweet potatoes and broth, cover and bring to a boil over high flame. Reduce heat and simmer for about 35 minutes or until potatoes are tender.

2. Transfer into a blender and mix until pureed. Transfer back into the pot, add coconut milk and heat for several seconds until heated through.

WATERCRESS SOUP

Servings: 4

Ingredients:

- **1 quart chicken stock**
- **1 medium leek**
- **1 teaspoon coconut oil**
- **1 bunch watercress**
- **1 large onion**
- **1/2 celeriac root, skinned and chopped**
- **Salt and pepper to taste**
- **Coconut cream, for garnish**

Directions:

1. In a pot, gently boil the chicken stock.

2. Meanwhile, in a skillet, heat a little coconut oil and cook onions, leek and celeriac for about 5 minutes or until tender. Reserve about a third of the mixture and pour the rest into the pot with boiling stock. Sprinkle salt and pepper to taste. Add the watercress and cook for another 2 minutes or until just wilted.

3. Using an immersion blender, blend the soup. Add the reserved vegetables and serve in bowls with a spoonful of coconut cream on top.

CHICKEN AND ASPARAGUS SOUP

Servings: 2

Ingredients:

- **1 bunch asparagus, trimmed, cut into 1/2 inch pieces**
- **4 scallions, parts divided, chopped**
- **2 quarts of chicken stock**
- **6 thin slices of ginger**
- **1 tablespoon coconut aminos**
- **1 pound chicken breasts, cut into strips**
- **2 handfuls of fresh baby spinach leaves**
- **Lemon wedges to serve**
-

Directions:

1. In a saucepan, combine stock, ginger, and white part of scallion; bring to a boil and simmer for about 5 minutes. Add asparagus and chicken, continue simmering for about 5 minutes. Mix in spinach, cook for another 2 minutes.

2. Equally divide the vegetables in serving bowls, add the soup and top with spring onions and garnish with lemon wedges.

ASIAN SHRIMP AND COCONUT SOUP

Servings: 6-8

Ingredients:

- **1 tablespoon coconut oil**
- **3 garlic cloves, minced**
- **1 tablespoon freshly grated ginger**
- **5 cups chicken broth**
- **1 cup snow peas, cut in half**
- **1 cup matchstick carrots**
- **1/2 cup coconut milk**
- **1 pound medium shrimp, precooked, tails re moved**

Directions:

1. Heat coconut oil in large saucepan on medium heat. Add garlic and ginger and cook for 1 minute. Pour in chicken broth, turn heat to high, and bring to low boil.

2. Add in snow peas and carrots, reduce heat to medium and cook for 3-4 minutes.

3. Stir in coconut milk and shrimp. Continue cooking for another 3-4 minutes or until shrimp are heated through.

CREAM OF BROCCOLI SOUP

Servings: 4

Ingredients:

- **1 tablespoon extra-virgin olive oil**
- **1 medium yellow onion, chopped**
- **3 garlic cloves, minced**
- **1 small head cauliflower, chopped into florets**
- **2 cups coconut milk, unsweetened**
- **2 cups chicken broth**
- **3 cups broccoli florets, chopped**
- **Salt and freshly ground black pepper, to taste**

Directions:

1. Heat olive oil in large saucepan over medium-high heat. Add onions and garlic and sauté for 2-3 minutes until onion turns translucent.

2. Add cauliflower, coconut milk, chicken broth, and broccoli. Cover pot and bring to boil. Reduce heat and simmer, covered, for 10 minutes or until cauliflower and broccoli florets are soft.

3. Pour mixture into blender or food processor and puree until smooth (may need to be done in two batches). Return to pot. Season with salt and pepper and simmer on low for an additional 10 minutes. Serve hot.

EASY CHICKEN, KALE, AND CARROT SOUP

Servings: 6-8

Ingredients:

- **1 tablespoon olive oil**
- **1 medium yellow onion, diced**
- **2 cloves garlic, minced**
- **5-6 large carrots, sliced thin**
- **2 boneless, skinless chicken breasts, cut into small pieces**
- **4 cups chicken broth, store bought or home made**
- **1 head of kale, chopped**
- **Salt and freshly ground pepper to taste**

Directions:

1. Heat olive oil in large pot over medium heat. Add onion and garlic and sauté for 2-3 minutes until onions start to soften.

2. Add carrot, chicken, and chicken broth to pot. Simmer for 35-40 minutes, or until chicken is fully cooked. Add kale to pot and simmer for an additional 5 minutes. Season with salt and pepper to taste.

Meat and Poultry

TURKEY AND ORANGE STIR FRY

Servings: 6

Ingredients:

- **2 tablespoon coconut oil**
- **2 cups roasted turkey, thinly sliced**
- **1 onion, sliced**
- **2 cloves garlic, minced**
- **2 teaspoon ginger, grated**
- **1 tablespoon orange zest**
- **2/3 cup orange juice**
- **¼ cup chicken stock**
- **1 large bok choy, chopped**
- **1 orange, segmented**

Directions:

1. In a non-stick pan, heat coconut oil on medium heat. Add in onion and cook for about 3 minutes. Add in garlic and ginger, cook for 2 more minutes.

2. Next, add in orange zest, orange juice, and chicken stock. Bring mixture to a boil. Then, add in slices of turkey. Reduce the heat to medium-low and simmer for about 3 minutes. Remove the turkey slices from the mixture and set aside. Add in bok choy and cook until soft.

3. Transfer the cooked bok choy in a bowl and layer the turkey on it. Serve topped with segmented orange.

CHICKEN WITH ROASTED SWEET POTATOES AND PARSNIPS

Servings: 4

Ingredients:

- 3 tablespoons virgin olive oil
- 1-1/2 tablespoons balsamic vinegar
- Sea salt and freshly ground pepper, to taste
- 8 chicken thighs, trimmed
- 1 medium-large sweet potato, peeled and cubed
- 4 medium parsnips, peeled and cubed
- 4 small shallots, lobes cut, peeled and halved
- 3 strips bacon
- 1/4 cup fresh parsley, chopped

Directions:

1. In a bowl, combine vinegar, oil, and salt and pepper to taste. Mix well to blend. Add chicken, mix to coat. Cover and chill to marinate for at least an hour to 8 hours, stirring occasionally.

2. Preheat oven to 425°F.

3. Evenly spread marinated chicken pieces on a rimmed baking sheet and drizzle marinade all over them. Arrange the parsnip, sweet potatoes, and shallots around the sides of the pan. Sprinkle with salt to taste.

4. Roast for about 30 minutes, basting the meat and turning veggies occasionally. Cook until chicken pieces are nicely burnished and veggies are tender.

5. Meanwhile, brown bacon in a skillet over medium heat. Drain on paper-lined plate to cool. Crumble and mix with parsley.

6. Transfer meat and veggies into another container, leaving much of the liquid. Toss with some bacon mixture, and plate. Serve, topped with bacon mixture.

PALEO CHICKEN IN A POT

Servings: 4

Ingredients:

- **2 ½ pounds chicken, quartered**
- **2 tablespoons olive oil**
- **4 large carrots, coarsely chopped**
- **1 bunch celery, coarsely chopped**
- **4 small spring onions, coarsely chopped**
- **1 quart water**
- **4 fresh sage leaves**
- **1 fresh rosemary sprig**
- **1 bay leaf**

Directions:

1. Preheat oven to 300°F.

2. In an ovenproof pot, heat oil over medium heat. Sauté carrots, celery, and spring onions for about 5 minutes or until tender. Pour in water and add chicken. Tie together rosemary, sage, and bay leaves together and combine with the chicken in the pot.

3. Cover and cook for about 1 hour inside the preheated oven. Uncover and broil for another 5 minutes. Serve with vegetables and broth.

CHICKEN, BACON, AND MUSHROOM SKEWERS

Servings: 6

Ingredients:

- 1/2 cup cider vinegar
- 1/2 cup coconut amino sauce
- 2 tablespoons honey
- 4 tablespoons coconut oil
- 4 green onions, minced
- 10 large mushrooms, halved
- 3 skinless, boneless chicken breast halves, cubed
- 1/2 pound sliced thick-cut bacon, halved
- 1 (8 ounces) can pineapple chunks, drained

Directions:

1. In a bowl, combine the first 5 ingredients. Mix well. Add mushrooms and chicken, cover and chill for about an hour to marinate.
2. Preheat grill at high heat and grease its grates.
3. Remove chicken and mushrooms from marinade and remove excess liquid; set aside marinade. Wrap bacon strips around chicken chunks. Thread on skewers, securing the bacon, along with mushrooms and pineapple in alternating pattern.
4. Meanwhile, boil marinade over high heat, then reduce heat to simmer for about 10 minutes or until volume is halved.
5. Grill skewers for about 20 minutes, turning occasionally and basting with marinade, until juices run clear and bacon turns crisp and golden brown.

FRIED CHICKEN WITH AVOCADO AND RED ONION SALSA

Servings: 2-3

Ingredients:

- **1 pound boneless chicken breast, halved**

Marinade:

- **3 tablespoons virgin olive oil**
- **2 cloves garlic, pressed**
- **2 tablespoons lime juice**
- **Sea salt**

Salsa:

- **1 ripe avocado, diced**
- **1/4 cup red onion, chopped**
- **2 tablespoons olive oil**
- **1 tablespoon lime juice**
- **Salt and pepper**
- **2 tablespoon coriander, chopped**

Garnish:

- **Red onion, sliced**
- **Lime wedge**
- **Cabbage, shredded**

Directions:

1. In a bowl, combine all ingredients for the marinade. Add chicken, mix to blend. Set aside for about 20 minutes to marinate.

2. In a heated pan, add oil and cook chicken over medium heat, until all sides turn brown and juices drip clear. Mix in 2 tablespoons marinade and cook another couple of minutes until glazed.

3. Meanwhile, in another bowl, combine all salsa ingredients up to lime juice, mix to blend, sprinkle with salt and pepper to taste. Mix in coriander.

4. Plate chicken and salsa, garnished with cabbage, red onion, and lime wedges.

Note: For a more colorful dish, use red cabbage and add some shredded carrots.

CHICKEN PICCATA

Servings: 4

Ingredients:

- **1 ½ pounds chicken tenders, boneless, skin less**
- **3 tablespoons coconut flour**
- **5 tablespoons olive oil**
- **3 lemons, freshly squeezed plus 5-6 slices**
- **2 tablespoons fresh parsley, chopped**
- **2 tablespoons capers, minced**
- **½ cup green olives**
- **Sea salt and freshly ground black pepper, to taste**

Directions:

1. On a chopping board, pound the chicken parts using a kitchen mallet to flatten to ¼ inch thickness. Lightly coat with flour.

2. In a large pan, heat oil over medium-high heat and cook chicken for about 2 minutes per side or until just browned and cooked through. Add lemon juice, capers, olives, lemon slices, and parsley. Lower heat, and simmer for about 3-5 minutes. Sprinkle with salt and pepper to taste.

BEEF AND BROCCOLI STIR FRY

Servings: 6

Ingredients:

- 1 1/2 pounds beef sirloin, thinly sliced
- 4 tablespoons coconut aminos, divided
- 4 tablespoons red wine vinegar, divided
- 3 tablespoons chicken broth
- 4 cloves garlic, minced
- 1 teaspoon arrowroot flour
- 1 teaspoon honey
- 1 tablespoon ginger, minced
- 1/2 teaspoon sesame oil
- 1 head broccoli, cut into florets
- 4 carrots, sliced diagonally
- 3 tablespoon coconut oil, divided

Directions:

1. In a bowl, mix 1 tablespoon each of coconut aminos and red wine vinegar. Add the meat, stir and marinate for about 15 minutes.

2. In another bowl, mix remaining vinegar, coconut aminos and chicken broth. Add honey, sesame oil, garlic, ginger, and arrowroot powder. Mix well to blend.

3. In a pan, heat 2 tablespoons oil over medium heat. Cook meat in a single layer for about 2 minutes per side until browned. Work in batches if needed. Set aside cooked meat in a bowl.

4. Add remaining oil into the pan, and cook the vegetables for about 2 minutes. Pour in about a tablespoon of water, cover and cook for another 3 minutes. Uncover, and cook until most of the liquid is gone.

5. Combine in the garlic mixture into the pan with the vegetables; toss to coat. Add the beef and mix until the thickened sauce coats everything in the pan. Serve at once.

GLAZED PORK ROAST WITH CARROTS, PARSNIPS, AND PEARS

Servings: 4

Ingredients:

- 1 (2-pound) center-cut boneless pork loin roast
- Kosher salt and freshly ground black pepper, to taste
- 2 tablespoons honey
- 2 tablespoons fresh sage, roughly chopped
- 1 cup carrots, peeled, chopped
- 1 cup parsnips, peeled, chopped
- 2 ripe pears, quartered, cored, stemmed, chopped
- 1 1/2 tablespoons olive oil

Directions:

1. Preheat oven to 400°F. Lightly grease a roasting pan.

2. Rub pork roast with salt and pepper. Place in the center of prepared roasting pan. Set aside.

3. Into a bowl, combine honey and half of the sage; whisk until blended and coat all over the top and sides of the pork. Meanwhile, in another bowl, combine vegetables and pears. Mix in oil and the remaining sage, toss well to coat. Add some salt and

pepper to taste. Place the mixture all around the pork; pour half cup of water in bottom of pan and roast for about 40 minutes or until inner temperature reads 145°F.

4. Put roast on a chopping board, tent loosely with tin foil and rest for about 5 minutes. Return vegetables into the oven if not yet fully softened. Serve pork sliced with veggies and pears at the sides.

HERBED RACK OF LAMB

Servings: 4

Ingredients:

- **3 tablespoons parsley, chopped**
- **2 tablespoons rosemary, chopped**
- **1 tablespoon thyme, chopped**
- **1/2 teaspoon onion powder**
- **2 garlic cloves, minced**
- **2 teaspoons sea salt (divided)**
- **1 (8-bone) rack of lamb**
- **1/4 cup olive oil**

Directions:

1. In a bowl, mix thyme, onion powder, parsley, rosemary, garlic, and 1 teaspoon of salt. Thoroughly coat the lamb with the herb mixture. Plastic wrap and chill for at least 2 hours to overnight. Take out from the fridge 30 minutes before preparation.

2. Preheat oven to 300 °F.

3. In a large skillet, heat oil over medium heat. Cook lamb for about 4 minutes fat side down until golden brown. Sear the other side for an additional 2 minutes. Put the seared lamb into a baking dish and roast for about 20 minutes. Let cool on a chopping board, loosely covered with a tin foil.

GRILLED BALSAMIC LAMB CHOPS

Servings: 4

Ingredients:

- **4 (1 ½ pounds) lamb chops**
- **1/4 cup balsamic vinegar**
- **2 tablespoons virgin olive oil**
- **1 tablespoon fresh rosemary leaf, finely chopped**

Directions:

1. In a bowl, combine vinegar, oil, and rosemary. Mix well. Add lamb chops, mix to evenly coat. Set aside for about 10 minutes to marinate.

2. Meanwhile, heat a grill plate, brush some oil and grill meat for about 5 minutes per side or until desired doneness is attained. May also be broiled.

ROASTED PORK WITH APPLES AND SWEET POTATOES

Servings: 6

Ingredients:

- **1 pound pork tenderloin, tied with cooking twine, if desired**
- **3 teaspoons coconut oil, divided, plus more for greasing**
- **2 tablespoons chopped fresh thyme, divided**
- **3/4 teaspoon sea salt, divided**
- **1/2 teaspoon freshly ground black pepper, divided**
- **2 tablespoons maple syrup**
- **1 tablespoon cider vinegar**
- **2 large sweet potatoes, peeled, thickly sliced**
- **2 large apples, peeled, cored, and cut into wedges**

Directions:

1. Preheat oven to 450°F. Position oven racks in upper and lower portions. Lightly grease a rimmed baking sheet.

2. Rub pork with 1 teaspoon oil, 1 tablespoon thyme, 1/4 teaspoon salt, and 1/4 teaspoon black pepper. Place on prepared baking sheet and cook in the upper portion of oven for about 10 minutes.

3. In a bowl, combine sweet potatoes, apple, and remaining thyme, oil, salt, and black pepper. Mix to coat. Spread mixture around the pork in single layer.

4. In a smaller bowl, mix maple with vinegar and drizzle half of it over the pork.

5. Return pork to the oven's lower portion and cook for about 15 minutes or until internal temperature reaches 145°F. Set aside, loosely covered with foil, to cool.

6. Make desired slices, drizzle with remaining syrup and serve with roasted apples and sweet potatoes on serving plates.

TENDER GRILLED PORK TENDERLOIN

Servings: 4

Ingredients:

- **1/4 cup virgin olive oil**
- **1 cup balsamic vinegar**
- **3 tablespoons fresh rosemary**
- **1 teaspoon chopped garlic**
- **4 slices pork tenderloin**
- **Salt and pepper to taste**

Directions:

1. In a zip-lock bag, combine pork with oil, vinegar, herbs, and garlic. Mix and chill for about 30 minutes.

2. Drain and discard marinade. Rub pork with salt and pepper to taste. Grill over medium-high charcoal heat for about 20 minutes, turning occasionally or until well cooked through.

3. Slice and serve.

Note: Other herbs can also be used such as sage and thyme. Garlic can be doubled for a nice aroma.

ASIAN CHICKEN LETTUCE WRAPS

Servings: 4

Ingredients:

- **1 tablespoon coconut oil**
- **1 pound ground chicken**
- **2 cloves garlic, minced**
- **1 medium yellow onion, diced**
- **¼ cup coconut aminos**
- **2 tablespoons rice wine vinegar**
- **1 tablespoon freshly grated ginger**
- **1 can (8-ounce) sliced water chestnuts, drained**
- **2 green onions, sliced thin**
- **Sea salt and freshly ground black pepper to taste**
- **1 head butter lettuce**

Directions:

1. Heat olive oil in large skillet over medium-high heat. Add ground chicken and cook, stirring, until chicken is browned, about 4-5 minutes. Drain.

2. Add garlic, onion, coconut aminos, rice wine vinegar, ginger, cook for another 2-3 minutes or until onions are translucent. Add water chestnuts and green onions and cook for another 2-3 minutes. Season with salt and pepper, to taste.

3. Serve by spooning a couple of tablespoons into the center of a lettuce leaf.

PORTOBELLO BURGER

Servings: 4 burgers

Ingredients:

- **8 Portobello mushrooms,**
- **3 tablespoons olive oil**
- **3 tablespoons balsamic vinegar**
- **1 pound ground beef**
- **1/2 medium yellow onion, minced**
- **Salt and pepper, to taste**
- **Toppings: lettuce, red onions, your favorite**

Directions:

1. Remove stems from mushrooms. Wash caps and pat dry.

2. Add olive oil to large skillet over medium heat. Add mushrooms and cook for 4-5 minutes. Flip mushrooms over cook for an addition 3-4 minutes. Remove from pan to plate. Sprinkle caps with salt and drizzle a little vinegar over each one.

3. In a bowl, combine ground beef with minced onion. Add salt and pepper. Form into 4 patties, about half-inch thick.

4. Cook burgers, either in skillet or on grill. Cook to desired doneness, flipping burgers once during cooking.

5. Place burger on mushroom cap, top with lettuce, onions, or desired toppings. Top with another Portobello mushroom cap.

BEEF AND VEGGIE STIR FRY WITH GINGER-ORANGE SAUCE

Servings: 4

Ingredients:

Marinade:

- 1/ 2 cup orange juice
- 4 tablespoons coconut aminos
- 2 teaspoons fresh grated ginger
- 3 garlic cloves, minced

Stir Fry:

- 1 tablespoon coconut oil
- 1 pound flank steak, sliced into thin strips
- 1 small yellow onion, diced
- 3 stalks celery, chopped
- 1 large carrot, cut into julienne slices
- 1 small bunch broccoli, cut into small florets
- Diced green onions, for garnish

1. *Directions:*
2. Combine marinade ingredients in large bowl. Add steak strips and mix so steak is fully coated in marinade. Cover and refrigerate for 30 minutes.
3. Heat coconut oil in large skillet or wok over high heat. Add on-

ion and stir fry for 1-2 minutes.

4. Remove beef from refrigerator, and drain, reserving the marinade. Add to beef to pan and stir fry for 2-3 minutes. Add onion, celery, carrot, broccoli, and marinade to pan. Continue cooking, stirring frequently, until veggies are tender and marinade starts to thicken.

5. Remove from heat. Top with diced green onion for garnish. Serve over bed of Cauli-rice.

SLOW COOKER SHORT RIBS

Servings: 4

Ingredients:

- **1 tablespoon coconut oil**
- **2 pounds beef short ribs, grass-fed**
- **Salt and freshly ground black pepper, to taste**
- **3 tablespoons balsamic vinegar**
- **1 tablespoon Dijon mustard**
- **1/2 cup water**

Directions:

1. Heat coconut oil in heavy skillet over medium-high heat until oil is hot. Add the ribs and sear on all sides. Season with salt and pepper.

2. Transfer ribs to slow cooker.

3. In a small bowl, whisk together vinegar, mustard, and water. Pour over ribs.

4. Set slow cooker to low and let cook for eight hours.

5. Serve with steamed veggies.

Seafood

PAN-SEARED SALMON ON BABY ARUGULA

Servings: 2

Ingredients:

- **2 (6 ounces) salmon fillets**
- **1 1/2 tablespoons olive oil**
- **1 1/2 tablespoons fresh lemon juice**

For the salad:

- **3 cups baby arugula leaves**
- **1/4 cup red onion, thinly slivered**
- **1 tablespoons extra-virgin olive oil**
- **1 tablespoons red-wine vinegar**

Directions:

1. In a bowl, marinate salmon with mixture of olive oil, lemon juice, and pepper. Let stand for at least 15 minutes.

2. In a non-stick pan heated over medium-high heat, cook salmon skin side down, for about 3 minutes. Loosen any sticking skin. Lower heat, cover, and continue cooking for about 3 minutes more or until just firm and skin is crispy.

3. Prepare salad by combining the arugula and onion in a bowl. Add oil and vinegar then season with pepper. Serve at once with the fish.

SMOKED SALMON AND SWEET-POTATO HASH

Servings: 6

Ingredients:

- **1 pound red-skinned sweet potatoes, peeled, cubed**
- **3 tablespoons olive oil**
- **1 pound leeks, chopped (white and pale green parts only)**
- **4 teaspoons fresh dill, chopped**
- **1 tablespoons orange peel, grated**
- **6 ounces smoked salmon, chopped**

Directions:

1. Preheat oven to 325°F. Lightly grease six 3/4-cup ramekins with non-stick spray.

2. In non-stick pan, heat oil over medium heat; stir and cook leeks and potatoes for about 3 minutes. Lower heat, cover, and cook with occasional stirring for another 10 minutes or until tender.

3. Remove cover, increase the heat and cook, undisturbed for about 5 minutes or until bottom of potatoes turn brown. Crumble potatoes and mix over and cook for another 3 minutes to brown the other sides.

4. Mix in dill, orange peel, and salmon. Equally fill prepared ramekins with the mixture; pat to compact. Bake for about 15 minutes.

MARINATED CALAMARI

Servings: 4

Ingredients:

- **1 pound medium-sized squid, cleaned, heads cut-off**
- **1/3 cup lemon juice**
- **1/3 cup coconut oil**
- **1 garlic clove, crushed**
- **1 tablespoon parsley, chopped**

Directions:

1. Cut squid into rings. Into a pan of boiling water, drop squid rings and simmer for about 10 minutes or until tender. Drain into a colander and transfer to a bowl.

2. In another bowl, whisk lemon juice and oil. Pour in the squid, mix, cover, and chill overnight.

3. The following day, mix in garlic and parsley, and marinate further for another 2 hours or more. Serve and enjoy with the marinade.

GRILLED WHITEFISH WITH OREGANO

Servings: 4

Ingredients:

- **1 1/2 pounds white fish fillets**
- **1 tablespoon orange juice**
- **1 tablespoon lemon juice**
- **1 tablespoon fresh oregano, chopped**
- **1/2 teaspoon sea salt**
- **1 tablespoon virgin olive oil**

Directions:

1. Preheat oven to 450 °F. Lightly grease a large baking sheet.

2. In a bowl, combine olive oil with the fruit juices, oregano, and salt. Spread fish fillets on the prepared baking sheet in single layer. Brush generously with the dressing and roast for about 10 minutes or until flaky.

3. Serve warm with some blanched Brussels sprouts or asparagus sticks.

Note: Use cod, haddock, or any white fish. Orange juice can be omitted. Fresh or dried oregano can be used. Oregano can be substituted with fresh marjoram.

BROILED HALIBUT WITH FRUIT SALSA

Servings: 4

Ingredients:

- **1 pound halibut fillets, about 1-inch thick, fresh or thawed**
- **3/4 cup fresh strawberries, chopped**
- **1/3 cup peeled kiwi fruits, chopped**
- **1 tablespoon fresh cilantro, snipped**
- **1 tablespoon orange juice**
- **1 teaspoon coconut oil**
- **1/4 teaspoon lemon juice**
- **¼ teaspoon black pepper**
- **Nonstick cooking spray (olive oil)**
- **Fresh cilantro stem (if desired)**

Directions:

1. Preheat oven to its broiling temperature. Lightly grease rack of a broiler pan.
2. In a large bowl, combine all fruits and set aside.
3. In another bowl, put fish fillets and drizzle with oil. Mix to coat. Drizzle lemon juice and sprinkle pepper to taste. Spread fish on prepared pan and broil 4 inches from the heat source for about 10 minutes, or until flaky. Flip once.
4. Equally divide fish on 4 plates and serve with the fruit salsa on top.

Note: Salmon fillets are an excellent substitute. Peaches or nectarines can be used instead of strawberries; apricots instead of kiwi; and apple juice instead of orange juice.

GRILLED MARINATED TUNA IN FOIL WITH ONIONS

Servings: 4

Ingredients:

- **4 slices fresh tuna, about 1-inch thick**
- **1/2 cup balsamic vinegar**
- **salt & pepper**
- **1 cup fresh mint leaves**
- **2 teaspoon dried oregano**
- **2 large onions, sliced very thinly**
- **Virgin olive oil**

Directions:

Preheat oven to 350°F.

1. In a glass bowl, combine vinegar, mint, salt, and pepper. Mix well. Add tuna slices, gently stir to coat. Set aside for at least 10 minutes.

2. Prepare 4 large pieces of foil; coat each inside of foil sheets with oil and line with sliced onions. Drain and discard marinade of fish. Arrange each of the slices onto the foils and cover with another layer of onion slices.

3. Fold foil over the fish and fold tightly to seal. Bake for about 10 minutes.

Note: The fish packets can also be grilled for about 15 minutes. Vidalia onions or sweet onions can be used.

CLAMS IN VEGETABLE BROTH

Servings: 4

Ingredients:

- **50 small clams in shell, scrubbed**
- **2 tablespoons extra-virgin olive oil**
- **6 cloves garlic, minced**
- **1 cup low sodium vegetable broth**
- **2 tablespoons coconut butter**
- **1/2 cup fresh parsley, chopped**

Directions:

1. In a pot, heat oil over medium-high heat and stir fry garlic for about 3 minutes or until lightly browned and fragrant. Pour in broth and boil uncovered until half has been evaporated.

2. Add clams, cover, and simmer until they start to open. Add coconut butter, replace cover and continue cooking for about 5 minutes until they are fully open. Discard unopened clams.

3. Transfer clams and liquid into serving bowls.

Note: Apple juice can be used instead of the vegetable broth.

CITRUS BAKED SALMON

Servings: 4

Ingredients:

- **4 slices lemon**
- **4 slices orange**
- **4 salmon fillets (6-8 ounces each)**
- **Salt and freshly ground black pepper**
- **2 tablespoons fresh dill, chopped**
- **1 tablespoon olive oil**
- **2/3 cup rice wine vinegar**

Directions:

1. Place lemon and orange slices, side by side, in the bottom of a large shallow baking dish. Place each salmon fillet across the citrus slices. Sprinkle with salt and pepper.

2. In a small bowl, combine dill, olive oil, and rice wine vinegar. Drizzle mixture over salmon fillets.

3. Bake in preheated 400 degree oven for about 20 minutes or until salmon is cooked through.

LEMONY GARLIC SHRIMP OVER ZOODLES

Servings: 2

Ingredients:

- **12 large shrimp, peeled, deveined, tails intact**
- **2 garlic cloves, crushed**
- **2 tablespoons olive oil**
- **1 tablespoon fresh parsley, chopped**
- **2 teaspoons lemon juice**
- **1 teaspoon lemon zest**
- **1 recipe <u>Zoodles</u>**

Directions:

1. In a large pan, heat oil over medium high heat. Sauté garlic for a few seconds then stir in shrimp. Cook for about 3 minutes or until shrimp starts to turn pink.

2. Mix in chopped parsley, lemon zest, and juice. Toss to blend.

3. Serve over Zoodles.

TILAPIA AND VEGGIES BAKED IN PARCHMENT

Servings: 4

Ingredients:

- 1 bunch asparagus, washed and trimmed
- 8 small carrots, peeled julienned
- 4 4-ounce tilapia fillets (could substitute cod, halibut, or other whitefish)
- 1 tablespoon olive oil
- 2 cloves garlic, minced
- Juice of 1 lemon
- 1 orange, sliced thin
- Salt and freshly ground black pepper, to taste

Directions:

1. Preheat oven to 400 degrees. Cut four 12-inch squares of parchment paper, fold in half.
2. In each packet place 1/4 of asparagus, 1/4 of carrots, 1 piece of tilapia, and 1/4 of garlic. Drizzle with olive oil, squeeze on lemon juice, and sprinkle with salt and pepper. Top with 1-2 orange slices per pouch.
3. Fold parchment paper over fish and vegetables. Fold ends on both sides and arrange pouches on baking sheet.
4. Bake for 12-15 minutes or until fish flakes easily and vegetables are tender.
5. To serve, cut through parchment paper and pull back to expose fish and vegetables.

Side Dishes

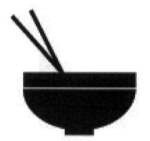

BRAISED LEEKS AND THYME

Servings: 4

Ingredients:

- **2 lb. leeks, white and light-green parts only, halved lengthwise**
- **12 small sprigs fresh thyme**
- **1 tablespoons dry white wine**
- **1/4 cup extra-virgin olive oil**
- **1/2 teaspoons sea salt**

Directions:

1. Preheat oven to 375°F. Prepare an 8-inch square baking dish by brushing lightly with olive oil.

2. Lay leeks, cut side down in single layer on prepared dish. Insert thyme sprigs in between leeks.

3. Meanwhile, in a bowl, whip wine, olive oil, and a tablespoon of water. Drizzle over leeks and thyme.

4. Sprinkle lightly with salt, cover tightly with aluminum foil and braise for about 45 minutes or until tender.

5. Remove foil and cook further for about 15 minutes until the leeks are browned. Remove thyme sprigs before serving.

BROCCOLI WITH GINGER

Servings: 4-6

Ingredients:

- **2 lbs. broccoli, cut in florets**
- **1 tablespoons fresh ginger, peeled, minced**
- **3 tablespoons olive oil**
- **½ teaspoon salt**

Directions:

1. In a large saucepan, boil salted water and cook broccoli, uncovered, for about 4 minutes or until just tender and crisp. Drain in a colander. Rinse with running water then transfer in a bowl.

2. In the same pan, heat oil over medium-high heat for about 30 seconds. Stir-fry ginger for about 15 seconds. Mix in broccoli, and cook for another 3 minutes.

ROASTED BEETS AND FENNEL WITH BALSAMIC GLAZE

Servings: 4

Ingredients:

- **3-4 large beets, peeled and cut into chunks**
- **1 stalk fennel, tops cut off and cut into chunks**
- **1 medium onion, diced**
- **1/3 cup extra virgin olive oil**
- **1/3 cup balsamic vinegar**
- **Sea salt, to taste**

Directions:

1. Spread beets, fennel, and onion in single layer on baking sheet.

2. Drizzle olive oil and then vinegar over vegetables. Season with salt. Mix with spoon until vegetables are thoroughly coated.

3. Place in preheated 400 degree oven for 40-50 minutes or until beets are tender. Turn vegetables every 15 minutes or so while cooking.

4. Serve hot or chilled.

ROASTED SPAGHETTI SQUASH WITH KALE

Servings: 8

Ingredients:

- **1 whole spaghetti squash, seeded, halved**
- **Olive oil**
- **Salt and black pepper**
- **2 bunches kale, stalks removed and torn into pieces**
- **1/2 whole onion, diced**
- **1 teaspoon balsamic vinegar**

Directions:

1. Preheat oven to 350 °F.

2. Place spaghetti squash on a baking sheet, skin side down. Drizzle olive oil on cut side and cook inside preheated oven for about an hour or until just fork tender.

3. Meanwhile, in a pan, heat 1 tablespoon oil over medium-high heat and cook onions for about 3 minutes or until tender. Mix in kale, sprinkle with salt and pepper, and cook for another 5 minutes or until kale is partly cooked. Remove from heat and set aside.

4. Shred the cooked squash using fork and put into a bowl. Mix balsamic vinegar with 1 tablespoon olive oil and drizzle over the shredded squash. Add salt and pepper; toss to blend.

5. Place spaghetti squash in serving bowls and top with sautéed kale.

ROASTED BALSAMIC VEGETABLES

Servings: 4

Ingredients:

- **2 cups butternut squash, cubed**
- **1½ cup broccoli florets, chopped**
- **½ red onion, chopped**
- **1 zucchini, chopped**
- **1 large garlic clove, minced**
- **2 tablespoon olive oil**
- **1 tablespoon balsamic vinegar**
- **1½ teaspoon fresh rosemary**
- **½ teaspoon sea salt**

Directions:

1. Preheat oven to 425 °F.

2. In a bowl, combine oil, rosemary, vinegar, salt, and pepper; mix to blend. Mix in the vegetables, mix to coat evenly. Evenly spread on a parchment-lined baking sheet and roast for about 50 minutes or until squash is just softened.

PARSNIP, PARSLEY, AND CAPERS WITH BACON

Servings: 4

Ingredients:

- **3 thick slices bacon, diced**
- **6 parsnips, about 6-10 inches long**
- **1 clove garlic, minced**
- **2 tablespoon fresh flat leaf parsley**
- **1 tablespoon capers**
- **Olive oil to garnish**

Directions:

1. In a non-stick pan, cook bacon over low heat for about 20 minutes or until browned.

2. Meanwhile, create ribbons out of the parsnip using a carrot peeler. Add these parsnip ribbons along with garlic into the pan with the bacon. Mix until fully coated with bacon grease. Cover and cook on low heat for about 18 minutes with occasional stirring.

3. Remove from heat; mix in capers and parsley until fully blended. Drizzle with some olive oil and serve.

TANGY ROASTED BROCCOLI WITH GARLIC

Servings: 6

Ingredients:

- **2 heads broccoli, cut into florets**
- **1 clove garlic, minced**
- **2 teaspoon extra-virgin olive oil**
- **1 teaspoon sea salt**
- **1/2 teaspoon ground black pepper**
- **1/2 teaspoon lemon juice**

Directions:

1. Preheat oven to 400 °F.

2. In a bowl, combine oil, garlic, salt, and black pepper. Add broccoli. Toss to coat. Evenly scatter broccoli on a baking sheet and roast for about 18 minutes or until fork tender.

3. Plate and drizzle lemon juice. Serve at once.

Note: Broccoli stems can be used too with the florets. Double the garlic if so desired.

STIR-FRIED CABBAGE WITH BACON

Servings: 6

Ingredients:

- **6 cups cabbage, cut into thin wedges**
- **3 slices cured bacon, chopped**
- **1/4 cup onion chopped**
- **2 tablespoon water**
- **Sea salt to taste**
- **1 tablespoon cider vinegar**

Directions:

1. In a pan heated over medium-high heat, evenly brown bacon for about 5 minutes or until crunchy. Set aside on a paper-lined plate.

2. Into the same pan with bacon grease, add cabbage along with the water and salt. Stir and cook for about 15 minutes or until wilted. Mix in bacon, cook for several seconds until heated through.

3. Drizzle with vinegar before serving.

ROASTED SWEET POTATO
WITH ROSEMARY

Servings: 6

Ingredients:

- **2 pounds sweet potatoes, scrubbed, cubed**
- **1 teaspoon olive oil**
- **1 dash fresh rosemary, finely chopped**
- **1 dash lemon juice**

Directions:

1. Preheat oven to 375 °F.

2. In a bowl, toss sweet potatoes with oil. Evenly spread on a baking sheet, sprinkle with rosemary and roast for about 30 minutes, turning once.

3. Drizzle with lemon juice and serve.

FRIED BRUSSELS SPROUTS

Servings: 4

Ingredients:

- **1 pound Brussels sprouts, whole**
- **5 tablespoons coconut oil**
- **4 garlic cloves, minced**
- **Dash of lemon juice, for garnish**
- **Sea salt, to taste**
- **Black pepper, to taste**

Directions:

1. In a pan, heat oil over medium heat. Add whole Brussel sprouts, stir and cook for about 5 minutes or until browned but not charred.

2. Mix in garlic and cook for another minute or until garlic turn light brown. Sprinkle salt and pepper to taste. Drizzle lemon juice. Serve warm.

Note: Add some shredded coconut along with garlic.

COLLARD GREENS WITH BACON

Servings: 4

Ingredients:

- **4 slices cured bacon, cut into small pieces**
- **1 medium onion, chopped**
- **4 garlic cloves, minced**
- **8 cups collard greens, tough stems removed and cleaned well**
- **1 teaspoon sea salt**
- **1 teaspoon black pepper**
- **1 1/2 cups low sodium chicken stock**

Directions:

1. In a large sauce pan, cook bacon until browned. Mix in garlic and onions and cook for about 3 minutes or until tender and browned.

2. Add collard greens and broth, mix to blend, cover and cook over medium flame for about 30 minutes or until tender.

3. Season with salt and pepper and serve warm.

GARLICKY ROASTED CAULIFLOWER

Servings: 6

Ingredients:

- **1/4 cup virgin olive oil, plus more**
- **1 large cauliflower, trimmed and cut into bite size pieces**
- **16 garlic cloves, peeled, lightly crushed**
- **1 -2 teaspoons fresh rosemary, minced**
- **1 teaspoon sea salt**
- **1/2 teaspoon black pepper**
- **Dash of lemon juice**

Directions:

1. Preheat oven to 450 °F.

2. In a bowl, combine oil with rosemary, salt, and pepper. Whisk to blend. Add cauliflower, toss to coat. Evenly spread on a baking sheet along with garlic and roast for about 20 minutes. Mix to flip sides, lower temperature to 350 °F and cook for another 20 minutes.

3. Served sprinkled with a dash of lemon juice.

ZOODLES

Servings: 4

Ingredients:

- **4 medium zucchini**
- **Salt and freshly ground pepper to taste**

Directions:

1. Using either your vegetable spiral slicer or julienne peeler, cut zucchini into long skinny noodles.
2. These can be cooked by stir frying in either olive oil or coconut oil for 2-3 minutes until tender or can be microwaved in a covered, microwave-safe dish for about 1.5 to 2 minutes.

CAULIFLOWER "RICE"

Servings: 6

Ingredients

- **1 large head of cauliflower**
- **Food processor or hand grater**

Directions:

1. Wash cauliflower and remove leaves. Cut cauliflower florets off of core; discard core.

2. Place florets into food processor (will need to be done in batches). Pulse until cauliflower is reduced to rice-sized pieces. Alternatively, use hand grater to grate cauliflower.

3. Cauliflower rice can now either be frozen for later use or cooked in a variety of ways depending on the dish.

Bake: Spread cauliflower rice on baking sheet lined with parchment paper and bake in 400 degree oven for about 15 minutes, turning once halfway through.

Fry: Heat olive oil or coconut oil in skillet over medium-high heat. Add cauliflower rice and sauté for 4-5 minutes. Season with salt and pepper.

Microwave: Place cauliflower rice in microwave safe dish. Cover and cook in microwave for 1-2 minutes, until tender.

ASPARAGUS WRAPPED IN BACON

Servings: 4

Ingredients

- **1 bunch asparagus (about 1 ½ pounds), ends trimmed**
- **2 tablespoons extra-virgin olive oil**
- **Salt and freshly ground black pepper, to taste**
- **4 slices bacon**
- **Lemon wedges for serving.**

Directions

1. Drizzle olive oil over asparagus spears to lightly coat. Season with salt and pepper.

2. Divide asparagus spears into 4 bundles. Wrap a slice of bacon securely around each bundle.

3. Arrange asparagus bundles on slotted broiler pan. Bake in pre-heated 450 degree oven 15-18 minutes, turning once, until bacon is crisp and asparagus is tender. Serve with lemon wedges.

ROASTED CARROTS WITH GARLIC AND ONION

Servings: 4

Ingredients:

- **1 pound baby carrots**
- **2-3 tablespoons extra-virgin olive oil**
- **2-3 green onions, sliced thin**
- **2 garlic cloves, minced**
- **Sea salt, to taste**

Directions:

1. Preheat oven to 400 degrees Fahrenheit.

2. In a bowl, toss carrots with olive oil, onions, garlic, and salt. Spread carrots in single layer on parchment or foil-lined baking sheet.

3. Bake for 15-20 minutes or until carrots are tender.

BABY ONIONS WITH BALSAMIC VINEGAR

Servings: 6

Ingredients:

- **2 pounds cipolline or pearl onions**
- **¼ cup extra-virgin olive oil**
- **¾ cup orange juice**
- **3/4 cup balsamic vinegar**

Directions:

1. Blanch onions in pot of boiling water for 20 seconds. Remove from water and place in bowl of ice water to cool. When cool, trim ends and peel.

2. In a large skillet, heat olive oil over high heat. Add onions and sauté for 8-10 minutes, until onion begin to brown. Add orange juice and vinegar to pan and bring to boil. Reduce heat to medium-low, cover, and simmer until onions are tender, about 6-7 minutes.

3. Remove onions from pan and place in serving bowl. Continue cooking liquid until it is reduced and has a syrupy consistency. Pour over onions and serve.

Sweets and Treats

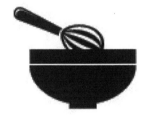

COCONUT DATE BITES

Servings: 4

Ingredients:

- **20 dates, pitted**
- **1 tablespoon coconut butter**
- **1/3 cup coconut flakes**

Directions:

1. Into the bowl of a blender, combine dates with coconut butter; blend until smooth. Form batter into golf-size balls. A little oil on the hands will help ease the work.

2. Roll the balls on coconut flakes and freeze for at least 20 minutes.

BROILED PEACHES WITH HONEY

Servings: 4

Ingredients:

- **2 peaches**
- **1 tablespoon extra-virgin olive oil**
- **1 tablespoon honey**

Directions

1. Preheat broiler.

2. Cut peaches in half and remove pits. Brush cut side of peaches with olive oil.

3. Place on parchment-lined broiler pan. Broil in oven for 3-4 minutes or until peaches are golden brown and caramelized.

4. Drizzle with honey and serve.

BAKED APPLES WITH HONEY
AND CINNAMON

Servings: 8

Ingredients:

- **2 teaspoons cinnamon**
- **½ cup honey**
- **8 large apples**
- **1 tablespoon lemon juice**

Directions:

1. Preheat oven to 375°F.

2. In a mixing bowl, mix together cinnamon and honey.

3. Core apples, Place apples in baking dish.

4. Spoon honey mixture into each apple. Drizzle a little lemon juice on top of each apple.

5. Bake in oven for 30-35 minutes or until apples are soft.

RESOURCES

Books

- *The Autoimmune Paleo Cookbook* by Mickey Trescott

- *The Paleo Approach* by Sarah Ballentyne

- *The Paleo Solution* by Robb Wolf

- *The Wahls Protocol* by Terry Wahls

Websites

- Chris Kresser – http://chriskesser.com

- Phoenix Helix – www.phoenixhelix.com

- Whole 30 – http://whole30.com

Index

A

acorn squash: Cinnamon-Squash Breakfast Bowl, 47
AIP. *See* Paleo Autoimmune Protocol (AIP)
alcohol, 13
allergies, 7
anchovies: Black Olive Tapenade with Tuna, 54
antibodies, 4, 6, 9
apple
    Baked Apples with Honey and Cinnamon, 140
    Banana-Apple Smoothie with Greens, 41
    Cinnamon-Squash Breakfast Bowl, 47
    Fruity Carrot Soup, 76
    Mixed Vegetable and Fruit Salad, 61
    Roasted Pork with Apples and Sweet Potatoes, 98–99
    Spinach Salad with Apple, 60
arugula: Pan-Seared Salmon on Baby Arugula, 108
Asian Chicken Lettuce Wraps, 101
Asian Shrimp and Coconut Soup, 80
asparagus
    Asparagus Wrapped in Bacon, 134
    Chicken and Asparagus Soup, 79
    Tilapia and Veggies Baked in Parchment, 117
asthma, 7
autoimmune disease
causes of, 6
    common, 5
    diet and, 3, 4–6
    increase in, 3, 4
    inflammation and, 4–5
    leaky gut and, 6–7
avocado
    Avocado-Berry Smoothie, 46
    Fried Chicken with Avocado and Red Onion Salsa, 89–90
    Grilled Chicken Salad with Mango and Avocado, 64
    Guacamole, 65
    Salmon Salad with Fresh Dill and Veggies, 63

B

bacon
    Asparagus Wrapped in Bacon, 134
    Chicken, Bacon, and Mushroom Skewers, 88
    Collard Greens with Bacon, 130
    Easy Bacon, Mushroom, and Kale Skillet Breakfast, 45
    Parsnip, Parsley, and Capers with Bacon, 125
    Pumpkin and Bacon Soup, 74
    Stir-Fried Cabbage with Bacon, 127
banana
    Banana-Apple Smoothie with Greens, 41
    Banana-Pear Breakfast Medley, 51
    Coconut-Banana "Oatmeal," 42
beans, 12
beef
    Beef and Broccoli Stir Fry, 92–93
    Beef and Veggie Stir Fry with Ginger-Orange Sauce, 103–104
    Portobello Burger, 102
    Slow Cooker Short Ribs, 105
beets: Roasted Beets and Fennel with Balsamic Glaze, 122
beverages, 19
Blueberry-Mango-Pineapple Salad, 69
bok choy: Turkey and Orange Stir Fry, 84
Bone Broth, 72
breakfast, 27
    Avocado-Berry Smoothie, 46
    Banana-Apple Smoothie with Greens, 41

Banana-Pear Breakfast Medley, 51
Broiled Grapefruit, 50
Carrot, Cabbage, and Peach Smoothie, 40
Cinnamon-Squash Breakfast Bowl, 47
Coconut-Banana "Oatmeal," 42
Coconut Milk Yogurt, 49
Easy Bacon, Mushroom, and Kale Skillet Breakfast, 45
Kale and Mango Smoothie, 43
Paleo Autoimmune Protocol (AIP), 48
Spinach and Sausage Breakfast Stir-Fry, 44
broccoli
Beef and Broccoli Stir Fry, 92–93
Beef and Veggie Stir Fry with Ginger-Orange Sauce, 103–104
Broccoli with Ginger, 121
Cream of Broccoli Soup, 81
Raw Broccoli Salad, 68
Roasted Balsamic Vegetables, 124
Tangy Roasted Broccoli with Garlic, 126
Brussels Sprouts, Fried, 129
butternut squash
Roasted Balsamic Vegetables, 124
Shitake Soup with Squash and Mustard Greens, 73

C

cabbage
Carrot, Cabbage, and Peach Smoothie, 40
Stir-Fried Cabbage with Bacon, 127
Calamari, Marinated, 110
candida, 7
cantaloupe: Mixed Vegetable and Fruit Salad, 61
carrots
Asian Shrimp and Coconut Soup, 80
Carrot, Cabbage, and Peach Smoothie, 40
Easy Chicken, Kale, and Carrot Soup, 82
Fruity Carrot Soup, 76
Glazed Pork Roast with Carrots, Parsnips, and Pears, 94–95

Greens Chicken Salad with Root Vegetable Dressing, 57–58
Paleo Chicken in a Pot, 87
Roasted Carrots with Garlic and Onion, 135
Tilapia and Veggies Baked in Parchment, 117
cauliflower
Cauliflower "Rice," 133
Cream of Broccoli Soup, 81
Garlicky Roasted Cauliflower, 131
celiac disease, 5
chicken
Asian Chicken Lettuce Wraps, 101
Chicken, Bacon, and Mushroom Skewers, 88
Chicken and Asparagus Soup, 79
Chicken Piccata, 91
Chicken with Roasted Sweet Potatoes and Parsnips, 85–86
Cream of Chicken Soup, 75
Easy Chicken, Kale, and Carrot Soup, 82
Fried Chicken with Avocado and Red Onion Salsa, 89–90
Greens Chicken Salad with Root Vegetable Dressing, 57–58
Grilled Chicken Salad with Mango and Avocado, 64
Paleo Chicken in a Pot, 87
chocolate, 13
chronic inflammation, 4–5
Cinnamon-Squash Breakfast Bowl, 47
Clams in Vegetable Broth, 114
coconut
Asian Shrimp and Coconut Soup, 80
Coconut-Banana "Oatmeal," 42
Coconut Date Bites, 138
Coconut Lime Fruit Salad, 59
Coconut Milk Yogurt, 49
coffee, 13
Collard Greens with Bacon, 130
Crab Stuffed Mushrooms, 62
Cranberry Vinaigrette, 56
Crohn's disease, 5
cucumber
Mixed Vegetable and Fruit Salad, 61
Salmon Salad with Fresh Dill and

Veggies, 63

D
dairy, 11–12
Date Bites, Coconut, 138
diabetes, 5
diet, autoimmune disease and, 3, 4–6
digestive problems, 7
dips and spreads
    Black Olive Tapenade with Tuna, 54
    Chopped Turnip Appetizer, 55

E
eating out, 27–28
eggs, 11
elimination diet, 10, 10–11, 25
endive: Greens Chicken Salad with Root
Vegetable Dressing, 57–58
exercise, 29

F
FAQs, 25–28
fats, 18
fennel
    Roasted Beets and Fennel with
    Balsamic Glaze, 122
    Strawberry Salad, 67
fermented foods, 18
fibromyalgia, 7
fish, 17–18
    Black Olive Tapenade with Tuna, 54
    Broiled Halibut with Fruit Salsa, 112
    Citrus Baked Salmon, 115
    Grilled Marinated Tuna in Foil with
    Onions, 113
    Grilled Whitefish with Oregano, 111
    Pan-Seared Salmon on Baby Arugula,
    108
    Smoked Salmon and Sweet Potato
    Hash, 109
    Tilapia and Veggies Baked in
    Parchment, 117
flares, 4–5
foods
    to avoid, 11–13
    to enjoy, 14–19
    reintroducing, 20–23

fruits, 15–16, 26
    See also specific types
    Coconut Lime Fruit Salad, 59

G
genetics, 6
gluten, 6
grains, 11, 22
Grapefruit, Broiled, 50
Grave's disease, 5
greens
    Banana-Apple Smoothie with Greens,
    41
    Collard Greens with Bacon, 130
    Greens Chicken Salad with Root
    Vegetable Dressing, 57–58
    Shitake Soup with Squash and Mustard
    Greens, 73
    Strawberry Salad, 67
Guacamole, 65

H
Halibut with Fruit Salsa, Grilled, 112
Hashimoto's thyroiditis, 5
herbs, 18–19
hormonal imbalances, 7

I
immune response, 4, 6
inflammation, 3, 4–5, 6
intestinal permeability, 6–7

J
joint pain, 7

K
kale
    Easy Bacon, Mushroom, and Kale
    Skillet Breakfast, 45
    Easy Chicken, Kale, and Carrot Soup,
    82
    Kale and Mango Smoothie, 43
    Kale and Orange Salad with Cranberry
    Vinaigrette, 56
    Kale Chips, 66
    Roasted Spaghetti Squash with Kale,

123
kiwi: Broiled Halibut with Fruit Salsa, 112

L

lamb
Grilled Balsamic Lamb Chops, 97
Herbed Rack of Lamb, 96
leaky gut, 6–7
Leeks and Thyme, Braised, 120
legumes, 12, 23
Lemony Garlic Shrimp over Zoodles, 116
Lettuce Wraps, Asian Chicken, 101
lupus, 5

M

mango
Blueberry-Mango-Pineapple Salad, 69
Coconut Lime Fruit Salad, 59
Grilled Chicken Salad with Mango and Avocado, 64
Kale and Mango Smoothie, 43
meal plans, 31–35
meats, 16–17
medications, 27
melon
Coconut Lime Fruit Salad, 59
Mixed Vegetable and Fruit Salad, 61
mood disorders, 7
multiple sclerosis, 5
mushrooms
Chicken, Bacon, and Mushroom Skewers, 88
Crab Stuffed Mushrooms, 62
Easy Bacon, Mushroom, and Kale Skillet Breakfast, 45
Portobello Burger, 102
Shitake Soup with Squash and Mustard Greens, 73

N

nightshades, 12
non-steroidal anti-inflammatory drugs (NSAIDs), 13
nuts, 12

O

oils, 12–13, 18, 23
olives
Black Olive Tapenade with Tuna, 54
Chicken Piccata, 91
onions
Baby Onions with Balsamic Vinegar, 136
Red Onion Salsa, 89–90
orange
Beef and Veggie Stir Fry with Ginger-Orange Sauce, 103–104
Kale and Orange Salad with Cranberry Vinaigrette, 56
Mixed Vegetable and Fruit Salad, 61
Turkey and Orange Stir Fry, 84

P

Paleo Autoimmune Protocol (AIP)
FAQs, 25–28
foods to avoid on, 11–13
foods to enjoy on, 14–19
getting started, 10
overview of, 9
phase 1, elimination, 10–11
phase 2, reintroduction, 20–23
summary of, 23
parsnips
Chicken with Roasted Sweet Potatoes and Parsnips, 85–86
Glazed Pork Roast with Carrots, Parsnips, and Pears, 94–95
Greens Chicken Salad with Root Vegetable Dressing, 57–58
Parsnip, Parsley, and Capers with Bacon, 125
Peaches with Honey, Broiled, 139
peanuts, 23
pears
Banana-Pear Breakfast Medley, 51
Glazed Pork Roast with Carrots, Parsnips, and Pears, 94–95
Pesto, Zucchini, 70
phase 1, elimination, 10–11
phase 2, reintroduction, 20–23
pineapple
Blueberry-Mango-Pineapple Salad, 69

planning, 10

pork

Glazed Pork Roast with Carrots, Parsnips, and Pears, 94–95

Paleo Breakfast Sausage, 48

Roasted Pork with Apples and Sweet Potatoes, 98–99

Tender Grilled Pork Tenderloin, 100

Portobello Burger, 102

processed foods, 13, 22

psoriasis, 5

Pumpkin and Bacon Soup, 74

R

radicchio: Greens Chicken Salad with Root Vegetable Dressing, 57–58

raspberries

Avocado-Berry Smoothie, 46

reintroduction phase, 20–23

rheumatoid arthritis, 5

Ribs, Slow Cooker Short, 105

romaine lettuce

Greens Chicken Salad with Root Vegetable Dressing, 57–58

rutabaga

Chopped Turnip Appetizer, 55

S

salads

Blueberry-Mango-Pineapple Salad, 69

Coconut Lime Fruit Salad, 59

Greens Chicken Salad with Root Vegetable Dressing, 57–58

Grilled Chicken Salad with Mango and Avocado, 64

Kale and Orange Salad with Cranberry Vinaigrette, 56

Mixed Vegetable and Fruit Salad, 61

Raw Broccoli Salad, 68

Salmon Salad with Fresh Dill and Veggies, 63

Spinach Salad with Apple, 60

Strawberry Salad, 67

salmon

Citrus Baked Salmon, 115

Pan-Seared Salmon on Baby Arugula, 108

Salmon Salad with Fresh Dill and Veggies, 63

Smoked Salmon and Sweet Potato Hash, 109

salsa

Fruit Salsa, 112

Red Onion Salsa, 89–90

sausage

Paleo Breakfast Sausage, 48

Spinach and Sausage Breakfast Stir-Fry, 44

seafood, 17–18

See also fish

Asian Shrimp and Coconut Soup, 80

Clams in Vegetable Broth, 114

Lemony Garlic Shrimp over Zoodles, 116

Marinated Calamari, 110

seasonings, 18–19

seeds, 12

Shitake Soup with Squash and Mustard Greens, 73

shrimp

Asian Shrimp and Coconut Soup, 80

Lemony Garlic Shrimp over Zoodles, 116

skin problems, 7

sleep, 23, 29

Slow Cooker Short Ribs, 105

smoothies

Avocado-Berry Smoothie, 46

Banana-Apple Smoothie with Greens, 41

Carrot, Cabbage, and Peach Smoothie, 40

Kale and Mango Smoothie, 43

snow peas

Asian Shrimp and Coconut Soup, 80

soups and stews

Asian Shrimp and Coconut Soup, 80

Bone Broth, 72

Chicken and Asparagus Soup, 79

Cream of Broccoli Soup, 81

Cream of Chicken Soup, 75

Easy Chicken, Kale, and Carrot Soup, 82

Fruity Carrot Soup, 76

Pumpkin and Bacon Soup, 74

Purple Sweet Potato Soup, 77
Shitake Soup with Squash and Mustard
Greens, 73
Watercress Soup, 78
soy, 23
spinach
Crab Stuffed Mushrooms, 62
Spinach and Sausage Breakfast Stir-
Fry, 44
Spinach Salad with Apple, 60
squash
Cinnamon-Squash Breakfast Bowl, 47
Roasted Spaghetti Squash with Kale,
123
Shitake Soup with Squash and Mustard
Greens, 73
squid
Marinated Calamari, 110
stir fries
Beef and Broccoli Stir Fry, 92–93
Beef and Veggie Stir Fry with Ginger-
Orange Sauce, 103–104
Stir-Fried Cabbage with Bacon, 127
Turkey and Orange Stir Fry, 84
strawberries
Avocado-Berry Smoothie, 46
Broiled Halibut with Fruit Salsa, 112
Coconut Lime Fruit Salad, 59
Strawberry Salad, 67
stress, 3, 23, 29
sugar, 22
supplements, 29–30
support, 30
sweeteners, 13, 22
sweet potatoes
Chicken with Roasted Sweet Potatoes
and Parsnips, 85–86
Purple Sweet Potato Soup, 77
Roasted Pork with Apples and Sweet
Potatoes, 98–99
Roasted Sweet Potato with Rosemary,
128
Smoked Salmon and Sweet Potato
Hash, 109

T
Tilapia and Veggies Baked in Parchment,
117
tuna
Black Olive Tapenade with Tuna, 54
Grilled Marinated Tuna in Foil with
Onions, 113
Turkey and Orange Stir Fry, 84
Turnip Appetizer, Chopped, 55
type 1 diabetes, 5

U
ulcerative colitis, 5

V
vegetables, 14–15
See also specific types
nightshades, 12

W
Watercress Soup, 78
weight loss, 26

Y
Yogurt, Coconut Milk, 49

Z
Zoodles, 132
zucchini
Lemony Garlic Shrimp over Zoodles,
116
Roasted Balsamic Vegetables, 124
Zoodles, 132
Zucchini Pesto, 70

FROM THE AUTHOR

I hope you enjoyed the *Paleo Autoimmune Protocol* and that it helps you achieve your health and wellness goals.

Please check out our other titles in the Paleo cooking series:

- *Primal Paleo Cookbook: Quick and Easy Paleo Recipes* - *Paleo Diet: Beginner's Paleo Cooking for Health and Weight Loss*

- *Mediterranean Paleo*

- *Slow Cooker Paleo: Healthy, Quick, and Easy Paleo Recipes for Your Slow Cooker*

- *Asian Paleo*

More Bestselling Titles from Dylanna Press

Primal Paleo Cookbook: Quick and Easy Paleo Recipes **by Dylanna Press**

Whether you're just starting out on the Paleo diet or have been eating Paleo for years, the **Primal Paleo Cookbook: Quick and Easy Paleo Recipes** is going to help you make delicious, healthy meals without spending a lot of time in the kitchen.

This book was designed for people who want to be able to get their meals on the table fast, without the need for a lot of special ingredients or difficult cooking techniques. These recipes feature fresh, whole foods that are cooked the Paleo way—without refined sugars, processed foods, or unhealthy oils. They're perfect for those days you come home tired from work and need to get dinner on the table without a lot of fuss, using ingredients you already have on hand. Or when you want to put everything into a slow cooker and then set it and forget it.

Included in the Primal Paleo Cookbook:

*More than 100 Paleo recipes
*7-day Paleo meal plan
*Delicious, easy-to-prepare Paleo breakfasts, Paleo lunches, Paleo dinners, and Paleo desserts

Primal Paleo Cookbook: Quick and Easy Paleo Recipes is a book you'll turn to again and again when you're looking for delicious, healthy Paleo meals.

Mason Jar Meals **by Dylanna Press**

Mason jar meals are a fun and practical way to take your meals on
the go. Mason jars are an easy way to prepare individual servings,
so whether you're cooking for one, two, or a whole crowd, these fun,
make-ahead meals will work.

Includes More than 50 Recipes and Full-Color Photos

In this book, you'll find a wide variety of recipes including all kinds
of salads, as well as hot meal ideas such as mini chicken pot pies
and lasagna in a jar. Also included are mouth-watering desserts
such as strawberry shortcake, apple pie, and s'mores.

The recipes are easy to prepare and don't require any special cooking skills. So what are you waiting for? Grab your Mason jars and
start preparing these gorgeous and tasty dishes!

The Inflammation Diet by Dylanna Press

Beat Pain, Slow Aging, and Reduce Risk of Heart Disease with the Inflammation Diet

Inflammation has been called the "silent killer" and it has been linked to a wide variety of illnesses including heart disease, arthritis, diabetes, chronic pain, autoimmune disorders, and cancer.

Often, the root of chronic inflammation is in the foods we eat.

The Inflammation Diet: Complete Guide to Beating Pain and Inflammation will show you how, by making simple changes to your diet, you can greatly reduce inflammation in your body and reduce your symptoms and lower your risk of chronic disease.

The book includes a complete plan for eliminating inflammation and implementing an anti-inflammatory diet:

• Overview of inflammation and the body's immune response – what can trigger it and why chronic inflammation is harmful
• The link between diet and inflammation
• Inflammatory foods to avoid
• Anti-inflammatory foods to add to your diet to beat pain and inflammation
• Over 50 delicious inflammation diet recipes
• A 14-day meal plan

Take charge of your health and implement the inflammation diet to lose weight, slow the aging process, eliminate chronic pain, and reduce the likelihood and symptoms of chronic disease.

Learn how to heal your body from within through diet.